The Sophisticated Shopper's Guide To Plastic Surgery

The Sophisticated Shopper's Guide To Plastic Surgery

Richard Jobe, M.D.

Illustrations by Elizabeth Callen

Robert Erdmann Publishing
Rolling Hills Estates, California

Published by Robert Erdmann Publishing
28441 Highridge Road, Suite 101
Rolling Hills Estates, CA 90274

Copyright © 1990
Richard Jobe, M.D.
All Rights Reserved

Printed in the United States of America.
890123456789

ISBN 0-945 339-04-6 (Hardcover)
ISBN 0-945 339-05-4 (Paperback)

Library of Congress 89-084444

To Andi, my wife, who is everything to me.

ABOUT THE AUTHOR

Dr. Richard Jobe is in private practice on the San Francisco Peninsula. He is a Clinical Professor at Stanford University where he has been on the faculty since1961.

As past president of Interplast, a charitable organization which sends groups of doctors and nurses to perform and teach plastic surgery in Third World countries, he travels extensively throughout the world.

In addition to the aesthetic surgery discussed in this book, his special interests lie in surgery for facial paralysis, eyelid deformities, and cleft lip and palate.

Dr. Jobe lives in Los Altos Hills, California where he and his wife share six young adult children and three grandchildren.

TABLE OF CONTENTS

PREFACE

This book was written with a purpose. It is a statement of my opinion which is, largely, shared by other real plastic surgeons. There are some, whom I respect, who will object to parts of it. There are others, in the main physicians who don't fit my definition of a real plastic surgeon, who wish to be considered plastic surgeons, who will object vigorously to much of what is discussed.

I have been a full-time plastic surgeon for more than 30 years. I have divided my time between a private practice and an academic practice at Stanford University Medical School where I have participated in the training of over 80 real plastic surgeons. I have spent over a year of my professional life performing and teaching plastic surgery in the Third World with Interplast and Care Medico. I have a great deal of respect for our specialty, and I am sorely distressed by what is happening in the name of plastic surgery in our country and in other parts of the "First World".

In the United States, in particular, the trends in law and in government have severely limited the ability of the medical profession to police itself as it once could. The result is that many people are calling themselves plastic surgeons who have very limited qualifications. For reasons of their own, they have done and are doing things to unsophisticated patients which would have a much better expectation for an excellent result if the patient had been referred, instead, to the real plastic surgeon in the community. There are now about 4000 real plastic surgeons in the U.S., so availability is not a problem, particularly for the elective procedures we will discuss here.

This book has two general subjects. The definition of the real plastic surgeon and something about the practice, and a selection of comments about the common procedures for which a sophisticated shopper would look. Plastic surgery involves many other types of procedures, but these are generally techniques which are referred to surgeons, as is the practice in other specialties. Plastic surgery is unique in that so much of it is in areas where people seek surgeons without the help of their own doctor.

Finally, I want to express my appreciation to the many friends, teachers, colleagues, patients and residents in training who have helped me to grow to my present place in life. They are all speaking in some way through this book.

R.J.

1

What Is A Real Plastic Surgeon?

The term plastic surgeon is both meaningful and meaningless. For those of us who think of ourselves as real plastic surgeons, it means that we are or will soon be board certified plastic surgeons. For others it means one has designated himself a plastic surgeon because he does some plastic surgery without undergoing the training that is a prerequisite to becoming a real plastic surgeon.

What is a real plastic surgeon? This should be the first question of the sophisticated shopper. As you will see there are several answers. This book will, in various ways, tell you what I and other real plastic surgeons believe you should seek.

How It Started

Plastic surgery became an identifiable part of medicine during the First World War when many troops were injured about the face as they fought in trenches in Europe. The fathers of plastic surgery, as we know it in the Western world, are mostly British wartime surgeons who were very occupied during trench warfare, and for some years after, in restoring function and appearance to thousands of injured faces. A few American surgeons participated during the war. One of the best known was Dr. Kazanjian of Boston. During the 1920s and 1930s, a number of the founders of American plastic surgery spent time in British plastic surgical centers. They brought home concepts learned from their English counterparts and began to train younger American surgeons.

Plastic Surgical Training: An Overview

The Board of Plastic Surgery

The American Board of Plastic Surgery was founded in the 1930s along with many other medical specialty boards. It is now over 50 years old and has certified over 4,000 plastic surgeons in the United States. The founders came from various surgical specialties, dropped their original flags, and became full-time plastic surgeons with an intense interest in training their professional descendants.

A real plastic surgeon, who has a certificate of the American Board of Plastic Surgeons, is a full-time plastic surgeon, who has graduated from an approved medical school. This must be followed by at least three years of training as a general surgeon (Many are also certified specialists in general surgery). Some may elect to take the basic training in orthopedics or ear, nose, and throat/head and neck surgery as the prerequisite to the minimum 2 years of full-time residency in Plastic Surgery. If the prerequisite of ear, nose, and throat or orthopedics is elected, the training in either of these specialties must be sufficient to qualify for certification in the specialty. Although many real plastic surgeons are certified in their prerequisite specialty, almost none practice their earlier specialty.

The Residency
The plastic surgical residency is concentrated in areas of restorative, reconstructive, and aesthetic (cosmetic) plastic surgery. The resident becomes an active participant in all sorts of procedures and aspects of patient care that involve healing, transfer of tissues, microsurgery, burn care, restoration of hand function, reconstruction of congenital deformities (cleft lip and palate), care of facial fractures, and reshaping of body parts (both reconstructive and aesthetic).

The Examination
All of this preparation leads to the inevitable examinations which must follow acceptance in practice in some community or institution, and the performance of a number of procedures which must be documented and defended under the scrutiny of distinguished members of the Board of Plastic Surgery. About 30 percent of the applicants fail this examination. Some take it two or three times, some never pass.

3

The Product

All of this preparation is an excellent basis for the development of a surgeon who has the knowledge and skills to handle and move tissues with considerable judgment and facility. Plastic surgeons who then specialize in any area of aesthetic surgery, seem always to be grateful for the fund of knowledge and experience they had in other parts of the field during their preparation. Certainly, no real plastic surgeon would refer a friend or a family member to someone without this background for an aesthetic or reconstructive procedure.

Other Plastic Surgeons

It is unfortunate that any doctor can call himself a "plastic surgeon" anywhere in the U.S. Because plastic surgery is fun and profitable, many people who have not had the training outlined above call themselves plastic surgeons. They usually are trained in another specialty and do a few plastic surgical procedures--sometimes well. Often they are learning to do the procedures. They frequently perform operations they have read about, but have little knowledge of the more desirable alternatives. They generally do not charge less than real plastic surgeons. We have seen some tragic results of this adventurous behavior and are not proud of some of our medical peers.

ॐ

I have a letter given to me by a dermatologist, sent to him by a retired dermatologist, whose stationary indicates he is a member of a board related to plastic surgery that I had never heard of. In the letter he offers to show my friend, in my friend's office, how to do several plastic surgical office procedures. The board that he claims membership in, is an example of a board established to dignify its members. It is not approved by the American Board of Medical Specialists which is the standard-bearing organization of all established medical specialty boards. There are a significant number of these offshoot "boards" with beautiful certificates designed to confound the viewer.

ટ્ર

Recently, after a discussion with another experienced plastic surgeon about some of the details of eyelid surgery, I said, "If after our years of experience, training, and teaching, we still find we are learning more about what we are doing, how audacious do our outside competitors have to be, to do what they do to patients with as little training as they have? Do you suppose they are smarter?"

"No!", he said, "The problem is that they don't know what they don't know."

ટ્ર

Of course, we resent it. Those who have participated in, and struggled through the rigorous training we've been talking about are still human enough to resent the behavior of doctors who assume our title without having done what we have to earn it. They, of course, feel it is their right, since it is not illegal. The commonly used titles, Dermatologic Plastic Surgeon, Oculoplastic Surgeon, or Facial Plastic Surgeon, are indicative of a surgeon of more limited plastic surgical background and training than that we have described.

In summary, the designation, "Plastic Surgeon" has many meanings, and the sophisticated shopper needs to look further.

2

Clubs

All human cultures have clubs or societies for lots of different purposes. They were probably first formed as an excuse to get away from the family. Now clubs are formed by groups of people with similar lifestyles, the same economic class and professions. These clubs have social, educational and defensive functions. The medical profession is riddled with them.

ᶓ

The intrusion of the government of any country into the private practice of medicine causes doctors to defend themselves in various ways. At the present, in the United States, cosmetic surgery is one of the few refuges without government control. Many physicians are inappropriately finding cosmetic aspects for their practices to derive an income that is free of these controls. Unfortunately, aesthetic surgery has become for some, a business serving the doctor rather than a profession serving the patient. This is, of course, one of the great disappointments and disillusionments we have experienced in the recent progress of medicine--the "cosmetic" response to the invasion of government into the economics of medicine. It is a great temptation, if one can do it, to develop a cosmetic element in one's practice in order to have a portion of his work and its resulting income outside of the control of the bureaucrats in various capitols.

As a result, there has been an eruption of organizations to house bands of individual practitioners of various qualifications who profess to be cosmetic surgeons. Each club has its bold certificate to attest to the membership and assumed qualifications of the person whose wall it decorates. Some of these documents are true evidence of qualification and experience, but others are clearly not what they seem. The profession has innocently been advising the public to look at the credentials on the wall. The truth often does not lie in the credentials--certainly not the whole truth.

Even regular doctors, general practitioners, internists, gynecologists, and surgeons are not informed or have been misinformed about the true content of "certification". These real doctors have better and more complex things to worry about. So the potential patient cannot safely rely on his "good old doctor" for an appropriate referral.

Further, it is the nature of cosmetic surgical patients to wish to keep their level of vanity from their family doctor "who might not approve." Referrals are, therefore, sought from hairdressers, friends, advertisements and the yellow pages. The names of the organizations used to imply credentials all sound appropriate. It takes a sophisticated patient to find out the difference. Unfortunately, the possession of a license to practice medicine is not a guarantee of integrity.

The Clubs In Some Detail

There is a sharp distinction between the phrases, "Board Certified in Plastic Surgery" and "Board Certified Plastic Surgeon". The latter, "Board Certified Plastic Surgeon", is used by physicians who have been certified by boards other than the American Board of Plastic Surgery. In other words, they are certified in another specialty, typically otorhinolaryngology/head and neck surgery, dermatology, general surgery, or obstetrics and gynecology. The desired effect is to mislead the consumer into believing the individual is a credentialed plastic surgeon. In effect, he would be, according to present law, credentialed as he has a board certificate. And he would be a plastic surgeon since all a physician needs to call himself a plastic surgeon is the desire to do so.

The American Society of Aesthetic Plastic Surgeons

Regular members of this organization must be full-time plastic surgeons, board certified as plastic surgeons, who have been in practice at least seven years and whose practice has been heavily involved with aesthetic plastic surgery. They must also have been recommended as ethical practitioners and accepted as such by their peers. This is the only national organization of real plastic surgeons which is exclusively involved with cosmetic surgery.

The American Association of Plastic Surgeons
Regular members of this organization are full-time plastic surgeons, board certified as plastic surgeons whose contributions to the specialty, academically or organizationally, warrant election to this limited membership group. Membership in this organization does not necessarily imply experience or interest in aesthetic cosmetic surgery but it is a measure of considerable acceptance by the surgeon's peers. Contact with a member of this organization who does not have an interest in aesthetic surgery will likely result in a reliable referral.

**The American Society of Plastic
and Reconstructive Surgeons**
Candidate and regular members of this organization are fully-trained, full-time real plastic surgeons. Regular members are board certified as plastic surgeons. A candidate member must be certified within seven years of completion of training or he is dropped from membership. Membership is also based on appropriate professional behavior. Not all members of this organization are involved in cosmetic surgery, but those who are not will tell you so, and probably assist you in finding the correct surgeon. This is the "union" of the full-time and fully-trained plastic surgeons in the United States. This society has a large membership of leading plastic surgeons throughout the world.

State Societies
State societies of plastic surgeons are generally subsections of the American Society of Plastic Surgeons. They have the same qualifications, are generally groups of real plastic surgeons, and because they are more local, requirements for membership are often more stringent than for the American Society of Plastic Surgeons. This is certainly true

of the California Society of Plastic Surgeons.

ᨑ

The above are the certificates you should find on the wall of your surgeon's office. There will be others, but these are the important ones.

These are not all of the organizations said to include surgeons skilled in cosmetic surgery. There seems to be a new one every month. Some are international and originate in other countries. Some provide the surgeon with credentials and others do not. The fact that an organization is not mentioned here means nothing. I have only attempted to give you examples of what you should look for, and to encourage caution in interpretation of the framed documents on the doctor's wall.

3

Should A Plastic Surgeon Advertise?

(Caveat Emptor - Let The Buyer Beware)

For centuries it has been gauche and unacceptable for doctors to advertise their services. It was with great reluctance that physicians began to advertise in the yellow pages upon their initial inception.

More recently, as the yellow pages have become what the telephone companies hoped they would become, we have felt it was a service to our patients to be discreetly listed where we were expected to be. For many doctors, dentists, and lawyers, all of whom have had the same traditional reluctance, advertising beyond the courtesy listing in the yellow pages is an anathema, an inappropriate behavior.

ઢ

A few days ago at the doctors' lunch table at one of the hospitals where I practice, the subject of physicians advertising came up. It was proposed that patients should be advised to go to doctors with the least advertising in the yellow pages because that is where the varsity team of specialists and generalists will be found. Everyone at the table agreed. None of these colleagues, of course, advertised their practices. Occasionally, one will find the "top" plastic surgeons in a community advertising, but my review of the yellow pages in communities where I know who is the "expert" confirms this general premise: Few plastic surgeons of substance advertise.

ઢ

The subject of advertising came up again at a dinner party recently. A colleague's wife sitting next to me said, "What will you do when everyone is doing it?" This is an interesting question to speculate about. At what point will advertising be a useless expense because everyone will be doing it? At what point will plastic surgeons be selected by some patients, not on the basis of the quality of their reputations or their performance, but because of the relative skill of their public relations consultants? And, at what point will the cost of doing business rise because the cost of advertising is driving it rather than the needs of patients? Surely the cost borne by the consumer will rise under the burden of advertising? I am told by my patients that the heavy advertiser in my community charges more than his peers.

ﻬ

In the last couple of months, I had two patients who came in with the same stated reason. They both had talked to their friends and doctors, and had gotten several recommendations for plastic surgeons to help them with their aesthetic objectives. When they had to choose among the several recommendations, they decided to go to the one with the least advertising in the phone book. Both arrived in my office. I would call both sophisticated; one a biochemist and the other an entrepreneur.

ﻬ

Since the Federal Trade Commission ruled that doctors, lawyers, and other professionals could not be prevented from advertising by their professional societies, hospital staff organizations and the like, there has been terrific pressure exerted on the younger professionals to advertise lest they miss out on their "market share" (an unhealthy term introduced to doctors and hospitals in the last decade by public relations people).

In the past it was traditional for physicians to make themselves known to other doctors and thus consumers, by visiting them in their offices and by being very available on weekends and holidays. Young doctors frequently joined a church, a country club and the local Cancer Society in a graceful effort to build a practice. This was a slow process unless he joined an established doctor, which had its own hazards. This style of subtle advertising by gently offering service has completely fallen by the wayside.

Professional Behavior
Medicine is a profession in which the physician should provide a service which represents his best judgment of the needs of the individual for whom he works without allowing his own need for profit to influence this. A good example is

the relationship between a surgeon and his patient. A surgeon becomes a businessman when he recommends an operation of questionable or no value to the patient, or when he suggests he perform a surgical procedure on a person when there are distinctly better trained and/or more experienced surgeons available.

The pressure on some plastic surgeons to promote their practices is great. The costs of medical school, setting up a practice, paying office staff and the material needs of a family (which have been denied through the long years of medical school) are some of the factors that drive physicians to seek the highest income possible. The effects of these economic necessities are seen in the advertising activities of many plastic surgeons. From seminars held by plastic surgeons for hairdressers (frequently where consumers seek recommendations for a plastic surgeon) to societies that assist the plastic surgeon in providing materials (such as brochures, pamphlets, newsletters and videotapes), the efforts by some plastic surgeons to advertise and maintain "market share" can be seen almost daily in our environment.

While aesthetic surgical services can be advertised in newspapers, salons and the yellow pages, not all forms of self-promotion are valueless to the sophisticated shopper. The doctor's brochure can be an important source of information. The purpose of the brochure is to tell you some of the things about the surgeon that you would probably want to know. Where did he go to school? What societies does he belong to? Has he written or presented papers to his peers that relate to your reason for seeing him? At what hospitals does he practice? It's my opinion that this brochure should be available only to patients in the doctor's office or upon request by mail. My wife recently found a pile of one of my colleague/competitor's brochures on a table at the local women's athletic club along with a few of his society pamphlets with his sticker on it. I thought this was a little pedestrian to say the least (probably some of the women did too, but others probably thought it was O.K. and will remember him favorably).

Doctors have very different attitudes about advertising. There have been, since the beginning of the profession, individuals who could care less about the attitude of the local medical and dental societies, or their peers. Almost universally, they have lacked the respect of their colleagues.

The final word is not out on the subject of professional advertising. Several recent developments have increased the competitiveness of the practice of medicine. Competition by its nature breeds advertising in our culture. Certain actions by the government to encourage medical school growth in the 1960s and 1970s have led to an oversupply of doctors. The grouping of physicians into clinics and health maintenance organizations (HMOs) and preferred physician organizations (PPOs) have taken the management of medical practice away from the doctors and given it to managers who are not limited by professional traditions. They are also under considerable pressure to produce patients for their groups--so they advertise.

ەۉ

Cosmetic surgery, now being done throughout the world by people of various qualifications, is a natural setting for advertising as the patient who wishes privacy and discretion tends to be more vulnerable to advertising than patients seeking care for an illness. Some of the advertisements suggested by some of the societies (See: chapter entitled Clubs) surgeons belong to, are carefully designed to imply expertise that doesn't exist. That's the reason why I've written this book, to give you, the sophisticated shopper, an edge in finding the right plastic surgeon to help you meet your aesthetic objective.

ەۉ

One of my more cynical colleagues, a contemporary, on hearing me criticizing one of our younger ex-residents for his aggressive advertising posture, said, "Well, Dick, when do you suppose you will start?"

4

Should A Plastic Surgeon Solicit Surgery?

What is proper behavior for a physician when faced with the option to suggest treatment to patients? What is right? The usual physician-patient role allows the doctor to advise patients of what he feels will be good for their health; whether it be medical intervention, behavior modification, or surgery. This is because the physician must accept responsibility for his patient's health, even if his patient would prefer not to hear the advice.

The plastic surgeon often sees a scar, deformity, or evidence of aging that he would like to improve by his best surgical efforts. The physician's responsibility in this case is different as the correction he would prefer to embark upon may have little to do with the health and welfare of his patient. In my training, I was advised never to suggest an elective aesthetic procedure to a patient which has not been first mentioned by the patient. Newer ideas about patient education fly in the face of this advice, but there are many circumstances in which this should be remembered.

It is dangerous to guess why a new patient has come to the office of a plastic surgeon. Frequently, the patient will have a large nose or other feature which begs for the services of the surgeon, but will wish attention to something totally unexpected and often seen as unimportant by the surgeon. Experience has taught me to understand what my professors tried to teach me--what is important to the patient is important, even if it seems unimportant to me. It often takes considerable restraint to remain silent when I have a great idea about how I can help a patient, but I have never regretted remaining silent.

Some of the most miserable patients I have seen are ones who have felt ill-served by plastic surgery because a procedure was suggested by a surgeon when they had had no particular prior concern about the offending feature. They had accepted a suggestion because they believed the surgeon was the "authority" on the subject and have regretted it. These people expected perfection in the end result and in the social effect of the result.

Every senior plastic surgeon has seen patients who had gone to an otorhinolaryngologist about earwax, a plastic surgeon about a minor scar, a dermatologist about a rash, or an ophthalmologist for new glasses, to find most of the visit occupied by a dissertation on the patient's need for a blepharoplasty, rhinoplasty or face-lift. Such solicitation techniques are actually instructed in some residency training programs. Some patients have become exceedingly annoyed by such manipulation, but some are not. Many people become cosmetic surgical patients as a result of such suggestions.

Not all full-time plastic surgeons feel as I do about this. Some, for example, think it is quite appropriate to suggest a chin implant to strengthen the lower face of some patients coming in for nasal reduction rhinoplasty. My feeling is contrary. People don't come to the plastic surgeon for the reduction of a nose because the nose is large, they come in because they are bothered by the nasal dominance, often for some complex reason the plastic surgeon will never hear or comprehend. I have never had a patient, who has not first suggested a chin implant, come to me after a rhinoplasty wishing for a larger chin. A small chin below a large nose always looks less small after the nose is reduced.

People who want larger chins are a select group of the people who have, and are bothered by, small chins. This too can change. I spent most of my late high school and early college days with my lower teeth held in front of my uppers because I thought my chin was too small. Sometime in my early 20s this changed. My chin didn't grow (it wasn't particularly small or large to begin with). I just stopped thinking about it.

Orthodontists have an increasing propensity to suggest surgical modification of appearance to their patients. They feel they have a license to change appearance as they are constantly doing it in connection with the straightening of teeth. There is a certain flat-mouthed appearance, the signal of a good orthodontic result, that is remarkably common in the American middle class where a crooked tooth is a sign of parental neglect.

I was on an elementary school board in Los Altos, California, in the 1960s. At graduation, I used to count orthodontic equipment in the embarrassed smiling mouths as the children got their diplomas. Never less than a third of the children were in braces and many had, no doubt, left their retainers out because they were "dressed up". Orthodontists are good for the expanding market of aesthetic cosmetic surgery because they feel they have a right to influence the appearance of their clients. They are encouraged constantly to do this as well by their colleagues, the oral surgeons, whose dental surgical training now often includes aesthetic cosmetic procedures. This includes, in many instances, rhinoplasty, face-lift and other classical plastic surgical procedures as well as manipulations of the jaws. The modern young oral surgeon is not satisfied to stay in the office extracting teeth.

Patients rarely come to a plastic surgeon asking "What can you do to make me look better?" They generally come with a complaint and a plan in mind. They have often done as you are doing, read as much as possible about it, and are coming in to see if the surgeon is a nice guy and if he agrees with their perceived needs. The exception to this is the older person who comes in saying:"What can you do to make me look younger?"

It is safe to say that the patient who comes to a plastic surgeon with a specific concern that the plastic surgeon can do something useful about is the patient who is most likely to be pleased at the end of the aesthetic, cosmetic surgical adventure.

5

Self Image, Psychiatrists, And Plastic Surgery

Recent psychologic and sociologic research has confirmed the obvious. Better looking people do better in the world. They get better jobs. Teachers pay more attention to them. They get more dates. They are expected to be nicer, kinder and more successful.

The question is, is it the looks, or, is it the improved self-image and self-confidence the looks provide? There is little doubt that being raised in the presence of, "Isn't he an adorable child?" in its thousands of forms, enhances the self-image which promotes confidence, security, openness, and a willingness to speak up.

There is also research which demonstrates without much equivocation that successful aesthetic procedures improve the appearance enough that disinterested observers have better feelings about and expectations of the surgery patient. Unfortunately, it is not possible to accurately predict the quality of the patient's own response to such surgery. It would be wonderful if we could anticipate correctly the effect of a surgical procedure on the patient's self-image.

Most of us don't like something about our faces or our bodies and wish we could change it. This even extends to dress. For reasons that relate to something in our past, we have a peculiar focus on a part of our appearance. I have two colleagues whom I have known since medical school who are both quite successful and confident people. One's shoes are always polished to perfection, front and back, and his trousers always look as if he slept in them. The other's shoes always look as if he worked as a cement mason, but he never sits without lifting his trousers to protect the seams from his knees. I often use this example to describe the peculiarities of self-concern about appearance.

This attention to such detail is the same reason that brings patients to the plastic surgeon for help. In many years of practice, I have examined thousands of women's breasts. Most would qualify for some plastic surgical alteration if the typical concerns expressed by the patients who come in for surgery were the required standard. Fortunately, for the peace of mind of half of the population, this standard doesn't prevail. Two million women have had breast augmentation, though--about one in 50 adult American women.

Many of us, probably all of us, have some "defect" that could be improved by an aesthetic surgeon if we had the proper concern, the nerve and the interest to have something done about it. Often these "defects" are coupled with a concern that arises from things in our past that focused our attention on it. An unkind remark, a sudden awareness of our profile, or the way we don't fit well in a swimsuit are typical causes of this type of concern.

Once we have focused our attention on the "defect" it is difficult to erase the concern. A plastic surgical procedure, if it is appropriate and successful, will ease this concern. This is the most rewarding part of plastic surgery.

The most frustrating thing for the plastic surgeon is the patient who comes in with a problem that is quite obviously damaging the self-image, but who is not open to any plastic surgical procedure. Often this is a situation where we can say the concern is out of proportion to the defect. We sincerely wish we could do something. Sometimes there simply is no way of surgically solving a perfectly reasonable problem. Or, sometimes the surgery is too extensive and has too many secondary problems.

Even more disappointing is the fact that there is really no one else who can help this patient. Psychiatrists have very little success in diverting a patient's attention away from a feature the patient sees as an anatomical defect. These people often have no other problem that could give them a psychiatric diagnosis. They just don't like a part of themselves. As a result, psychiatric help is generally not available or, if available, useless.

When the concern is something like a child with a cleft lip scar or a major defect in the class of an anomaly, it is often helpful for the child to meet people who have succeeded despite a similar problem. In this case, group therapy, if available for this type of problem, is helpful.

A very wise and experienced plastic surgeon, Robert Mills, devised a scale a number of years ago where he compared the magnitude of the plastic surgical problem to the magnitude of the patient's concern about the problem. He found that the patient with the smaller problem and the greater concern about it is the most difficult to please. And, it is true that the patient with appropriate concern for even a severe problem is more likely to be satisfied with the effort. Occasionally, concern for problems of appearance are outgrown or worn out.

Concern and awareness of self-image problems on the part of the patient is just one of the considerations the plastic surgeon takes into account when he consults with a patient. The psychological state of the patient seeking plastic surgery is one of the more interesting aspects of the profession.

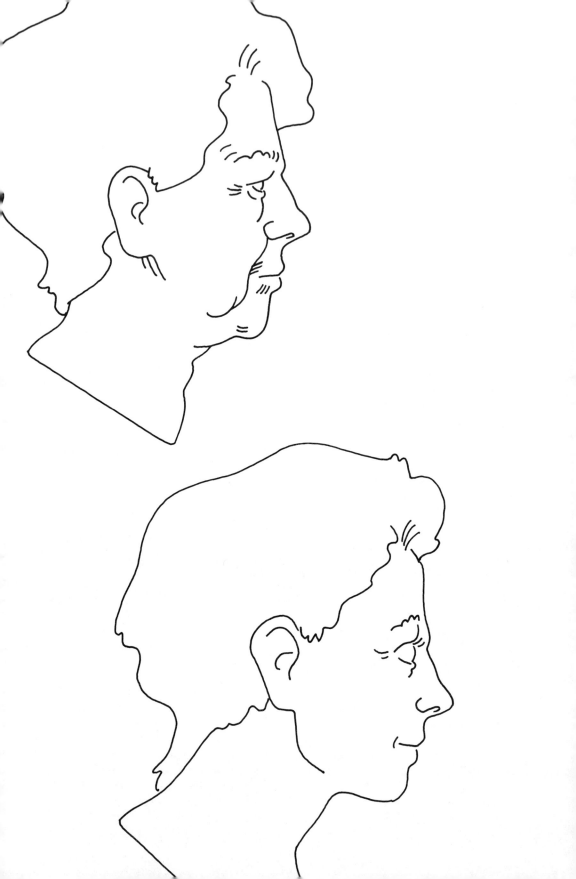

6

My Patients
Want To
Look Rested

I was sitting in a meeting next to my mentor, Max Pegram, who has a very successful and select plastic surgery practice in Los Angeles. We were listening to some of the experts talk about a new procedure that emphasized dissecting under the muscle in face-lifts. Looking at the photographic results of this new surgery, one was struck by the extreme tightness of the faces. This was an aesthetic meeting and all the masters of the plastic surgery art were there. I said to Max, "Are you doing these things?" His reply, in his unmistakable Mississippi accent was, "Why, hell no, Richard, my patients want to look rested, not changed."

The Aging Process.
Anyone who is considering a face-lift should know about the aging process: how it is affected by external elements, and how aging affects healing.

There are several factors that cause individuals to age in different ways. We begin to age at about the same time we finish puberty, but it isn't very evident then. Aging has a lot to do with skin thickness and elasticity. These two variables are part of what makes our faces look different from one another. The thickness or elasticity of our skin is determined by heredity.

Cutaneous aging comes in several types. In each person different features of aging are dominant creating differences in apparent age. It is difficult to judge the age of any mature individual because people age in very diverse ways. The most consistent occurrence in aging is the gradual expansion of the skin area. This is accompanied by the loss of elasticity in the skin (the kind of elasticity that makes rubber bands spring back to their original shape) which happens bit by bit. The rates of expansion and loss of elasticity are very individual. In addition, there is expansion of the ligamentous structures that hold the muscle and skin to the facial skeleton. This expansion allows the skin to appear to fall away from the skeleton making the sag visible when one looks down

30

into a mirror.

The sag looks much better when lying on one's back looking up into a mirror. In this position the extra skin can be felt in front of the ears. This is what I call "the undertakers advantage." When Grandmother is in the coffin, her sag is gone. It's in front of her ears. She looks better than she has in years because she has always been up and about for you. In fact, for the sophisticated shopper, it is possible to get an idea of what a face-lift will do for you by looking into a mirror while lying flat on your back.

How To Age Quickly.
The fundamental rate of aging is established genetically, and there is little we can do about our choice of parents. We have little opportunity to keep the aging process from happening, but we can make it happen sooner! There is no doubt that the ultraviolet rays in sunshine alter the architecture of the skin. In youth, the collagen and the elastic tissue have a well-organized structure. (It has the same three dimensional lacy structure we see when we cut or tear leather.) In the repeatedly tanned and exposed face or back of hand the structure looks like jello under the microscope, and such skin has no rubber left at all.

Sunshine and tanning booths both contribute to aging as well as speeding up the appearance of skin cancers and melanoma in those that are genetically predisposed to these problems.

Smoking, drinking alcohol, and a general lack of good health are all reputed to speed up the appearance of aging. There is not much researched data on this, but most plastic surgeons share this belief.

In women, the lack of estrogen also hastens the aging process. Some women seem to age overnight when they experience menopause. There are observed changes in the skin and mucous membranes that probably make one appear to age earlier. The use of estrogens is less controversial than it was a few years ago. I don't like to get into arguments with women's doctors, but I agree with a gynecologist/endocrinologist colleague that menopause is a deficiency state, and the deficient substance is estrogen. I am always a little relieved when the woman who wants to look younger is on estrogens. I have the belief that if she is, her face-lift will last longer.

Healing and Aging

In my experience, healthy people always heal. Those who are not healthy take much longer to heal. Smoking is the most common cause of wound healing problems in otherwise healthy people. This is because smoking diminishes the arterial blood supply of the skin and, thus, reduces the temperature of the skin and the nutrition necessary for healing.

Surgery does the same thing. People can recover from the surgical insult to their skin circulation, but not if the circulation is also being hindered by smoking. Of course, this is not always true; nothing is always true. But, we won't knowingly take the risk for cosmetic procedures under these conditions.

Children heal aggressively with lots of scar, particularly during growth spurts. Their rubber tight skin pulls on their wounds which defend against the pull by aggressive scarring. Adults heal well, with a little less strength in the scar than children. Adults don't scar as badly as children. Scars are often almost invisible in the elderly because the elasticity of the skin is no longer pulling against the scar.

What Is a Face-Lift?

A face-lift is technically called a meloplasty or rhytidectomy. These are translated "face plastic" and "wrinkle removal," respectively. The operation consists, principally, of removal of enough skin to make the face look younger. The techniques are fundamentally similar in that the skin is removed from the sides of the forehead, from in front of the ears and from the upper back of the neck and behind the ears. The connections between the skin and the muscle, and the connections between the muscles of

32

expression and the skeleton and other deeper structures, must be loosened enough to allow a graceful change. Precisely how this is done is, properly, an individual matter and the techniques of dissection to achieve the best result will vary from case to case depending upon the preoperative condition and the objectives of the surgery. One of the characteristics of the cookbook surgeon, as I call him, is the tendency to do this operation almost the same in every patient. The skilled aesthetic surgeon varies his techniques greatly as different problems are presented by the patients who do not, as we have discussed, age the same. I use the term "cookbook" because I think it applies to surgeons who have a limited repertoire of cosmetic operations without the surgical breadth to modify them as is needed to get the optimal result. It is like having a souffle made by a bride reading *The Joy Of Cooking*, or a chef at the Waldorf.

The SMAS
The subcutaneous muscular aponeurotic system (SMAS) is the combination of muscle and fibrous tissue that is immediately below the fat beneath the skin of the face and neck. Beneath the SMAS is a space that becomes quite dissectible along with age. It is the motion between the inner and outer walls of this surgically vague space that contributes the movement of facial tissues in response to gravity that we all call sagging or jowls.

In the past 15 years there has been a growing interest in the SMAS as something to be altered in the process of a face-lift. In the older face-lifting procedures, the skin was dissected from the layer we call the SMAS and the lift was done entirely above the superficial muscles and fibrous tissue; the space below the SMAS was never entered. A few years ago, in an effort to improve the results of face-lifts and perhaps to make them more lasting, dissection beneath the SMAS, to pull back and anchor the muscle, became a popular addition to the face-lift procedure. The result was, in many instances, face-lifts that

are tight and conspicuous, but for some of the plastic surgeon's clientele, this is desirable.

With time and experience, the aggressive manipulation of the SMAS in face-lifting is reserved for those
patients who want to be changed in appearance at the
time of their face-lift. But, even in the patient who wants
to look rested, some tightening of the SMAS is appropriate.

A Few More Details.

In youth, the eyebrows are more or less horizontal. The
part of the brow toward the center of the forehead is supported by the muscle of the forehead. The sides of the
brow are not supported by muscles so that the gradual
expansion of skin with age allows the sides of the brow to
fall. So the brows appear more as arches than as the relatively straight lines of youth. A face-lift, these days, should
extend far enough up the side of the forehead to provide a
compensation for the drooping side of the brow.

The hairline at the temple must move back if a face-
lift is done in the hair. Some of the elegant older ladies of
the stage, screen, arts, politics, and society no longer have
hair in front of their ears because of repeated face-lifts. In
some people this is preferred, but if a person has an ample
forehead it is often wise to do the surgery in front of the
hair. I often perform repeat face-lifts in this manner. The
closure of the wound must be meticulous. There is always a
scar, hopefully a fine one. Some people just don't heal well.
Anyway, hardly anyone looks at that part of the face. It
doesn't participate in expression.

Anesthesia For Face-Lifts

Most face-lifts in the United States are done under local
anesthesia with sedation. Most face-lifts in Britain are done
under general anesthesia with an anesthesiologist in atten-
dance. I personally don't care whether or not a patient
wants to be put to sleep for the surgery, but most patients
in the U.S. expect it to be done under local anesthesia.
There is certainly less risk involved, it also costs less and

recovery is a bit faster. The operation actually takes a little longer and requires a bit more energy on the part of the surgeon because he must manage the sedation and pain relief as well as the technical aspects of the operation.

Typically, the patient is given oral or intramuscular sedation at the outset. An intravenous solution is started and this route is used for further sedation to prevent restlessness, pain, or anxiety. The common drugs used at the moment are relatives of Valium and morphine. They are too numerous to mention here; each surgeon has preferred methods which are reliable. The objective is to keep the patient comfortable and have him alert enough to be able to go home a couple of hours after the surgery.

Ambulatory Surgery
Most surgery for aging is done on an outpatient basis, often in an operating room in the surgeon's office or a nearby surgical center. Most patients go home, though they should have someone with them for the first night. In some situations arrangements can be made for patients to go to recovery centers, or even hotels specifically designed for recovering aesthetic surgical patients. Hospitalization overnight is often appropriate for the patient who has high blood pressure or other medical problems. With modern anesthesia, it is even practical for patients who have had procedures under general anesthetic to go home a couple of hours after surgery.

Disappointments
We all live in the fantasy that we look half-way between the truth and our high school graduation pictures. If a face-lift is effective, it will make the patient look much like his fantasy. As a result, it is common for patients to look in the mirror a couple of months after the surgery and say, "I look just like I used to. Why did I have the operation?" This is why we take preoperative pictures and one of the reasons why the fee is collected in advance. Despite this common feeling, most patients are grateful that they had

the operation.

After a cosmetic surgical procedure, most patients inspect themselves in greater detail then they ever had before. They will, for example, become aware for the first time of the asymmetry or differences of the sides of the face we all have. This is often perplexing and is another reason we take preoperative pictures.

Complications

Face-lifts have the usual hazards of surgery such as the possibility of infection, bleeding and poor healing. Infection is rare and can usually be treated with appropriate antibiotics if it occurs. Infection is so rare that most surgeons don't use prophylactic antibiotics for face-lifts.

Bleeding is universal and usually shows with black eyes and other bruises. More excessive bleeding was much more common when we didn't know that aspirin was a common cause of postoperative and intraoperative bleeding. We now advise our patients to avoid aspirin for 10 days prior to surgery, and we see less of this annoying complication. Nonetheless, there is the occasional patient who will bleed enough to cause a collection of blood under the skin flaps which must be removed. Occasionally, the bleeding is so severe that the wound must be reopened in an operating room and the bleeding vessel found and stopped. For this reason we ask patients to avoid strain or stress for 10 days after the surgery.

Nerve Injury

All patients who have face-lifts will have some numbness around the ears which is noticeable for a time after surgery. Sensory nerves must be divided in the process of the dissection.

There is some re-growth of the nerves which improves the situation and the brain adjusts to the change so it isn't noticed after a time. As a result, it is rarely a problem.

Injury to branches of the facial nerve, the one that

moves the muscles of expression, is rare but cannot be guaranteed against. The vulnerable branches are those that raise the eyebrow or pull down the corner of the mouth. These branches are very close to the area of the surgery and they can be injured by stretching, clamping bleeding points or vessels next to them, cauterizing bleeding points next to them, or they can be cut in dissection. One of the reasons you want a well-trained and experienced surgeon is to avoid these rare injuries, but they can still happen with an expert plastic surgeon. These injuries are usually temporary and self-correct in a couple of months, but some can remain permanent. The deformity is not grotesque, but can be annoying. In my career, I can recall injuring three of these branches. The patients all recovered, fortunately.

How Long Will It Last?
Since some skin is removed from the face, only the skin that is left remains to age. So after the surgery one never looks as old as he would have appeared at the age he is. Unfortunately we have no way of preventing the aging process and as a result, eventually the patient looks as he did when the face-lift was first performed. The time it takes for this to happen is variable just as the aging process itself is variable, and for the same reasons. It usually takes between five and seven years to age to the preoperative state, though, some lucky people take longer and the unlucky ones may revert in less time.

A few patients with very heavy drooping skin of the cheeks and neck will require a second procedure within a few months of the first. This is not a second face-lift, but a completion of the first one.

Repeat Face-Lift?
Some people are concerned that if they have a face-lift, they will have to have another. This is not true. The result of a face-lift is permanent in that you will always look better than you would have at the age you are. Unfortunately,

the aging process continues and eventually, you will look as you did when you had the face-lift. At this point, you may say, "I don't need to look like this. I think I'll do it again." Having a face-lift gets you used to the idea. There is such a thing as too many face-lifts. There are women in the theatrical world who have had enough of them that it is obvious that they have been pulled too much in the only directions one can pull in these procedures. But, they knew what they were getting into and have accepted this trade-off, although, they do sometimes give the operation a bad name.

Other Procedures That Compliment A Face-Lift
It is fairly common to perform additional surgeries such as a brow-lift and blepharoplasty (eye lid plasty) at the same time as a face-lift. There is no particular reason not to combine these procedures, but there is a limit to the length of time a patient can be kept comfortable on an operating table, so some discretion must be exercised.

The Brow-Lift.
Becoming more popular and more frequently done, the brow-lift adds an hour to a face-lift. It is warranted when the brow droop is quite conspicuous, when the horizontal lines of the forehead call for correction, or when the vertical lines between the brows are a source of concern. The face-lift incisions are extended from the temples over the top of the forehead a bit behind the hairline so the scar can't be seen. Skin is normally removed to lift and tighten the forehead. The skin and muscle usually is turned down and the frowning muscle is removed or altered. Sometimes the vertical muscle is divided or partially removed to diminish wrinkles and animation. The brow can be loosened from its attachments to the skull and raised more effectively than through a face-lift alone. In people with higher foreheads, the brow-lift is rarely done below the hairline--the scar is likely to be a problem as healing is not the best here.

Often baggy upper lids are much relieved by a brow-lift. Unfortunately some patients look surprised after this brow-lift, but the lift generally relaxes after a time. Some surgeons' patients look more surprised than others, unfortunately.

&

Earlier attempts to raise the brow in cosmetic surgery were done by taking a strip of skin just above the brow to lift the brow. Regrettably, the result was a brow with a conspicuously sharp upper edge. The scars from this procedure were also less than ideal. The upper brow hair diminishes as the forehead begins. In nature this is not a sharp line.

From this "supra brow" procedure evolved the mid-forehead brow-lift, which is an acceptable but rarely used procedure. This is for the person known to scar favorably, who has a high forehead and a low eyebrow. A selected bit of skin is removed above the brows to raise them. The scar is usually remarkably inconspicuous, is in the correct line, and doesn't rearrange the shape of the brow itself. This type of surgery is more useful in males.

Larger Cheekbones?
One of the more recent additions to the face-lifting world is the use of prosthetic cheekbones for those who have flat cheeks and wish to enhance them. This procedure can be done without the face-lift and is often done on younger people. It is also performed as an accessory to surgery for the aging face.

The popular prostheses are of a material called Proplast, a porous plastic, but silicone has also been used. A few American surgeons have gained expertise with this modification.

The latest extension of face-lifting, comes, I believe, from the father of craniofacial surgery in Paris, Dr. Paul Tessier, who has initiated a procedure in which the soft tissues of the face are detached from the skull and elevated in the usual direction of the face-lift. The result is said to be most dramatic. How common this will become, or whether it will stay in style has yet to be determined.

Liposuction and Face-lifts

The use of liposuction to remove fat from a double chin during a face-lift is common. It is a very useful instrument for this purpose. It is also used occasionally to reduce fat cheeks where this is a desired objective.

હ

Face-lifting is part of the reconstruction of some facial disease and deformity. It is a standard part of the reconstruction of patients who have paralysis of the face, of neurofibromatosis (Elephant Man Disease) and other conditions. The youngest patient on whom I have done a face-lift was an 11-year-old girt whose face had been stretched out of shape by a blood vessel tumor of the type that goes away after infancy.

Proper face-lifting surgery, done to achieve the best possible result with respect for the patient's wishes, requires skill and great flexibility of approach. It is another procedure where experience and training are the details the sophisticated shopper should look for. Again, most patients who elect to have the surgery are grateful that they did.

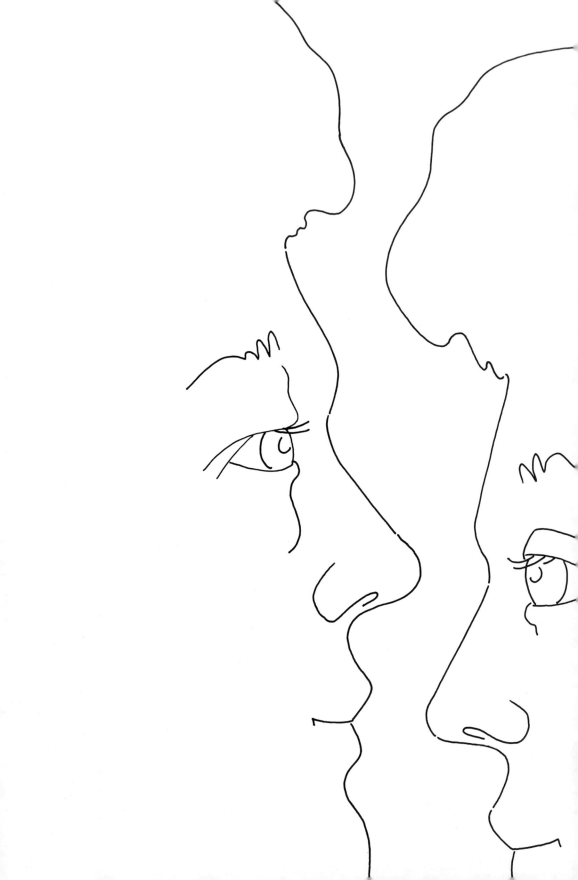

7

For Better
Looking And
Better Seeing Eyes

The thin skin of the eyelids is often the first part of the face to show that time is passing. The principal problem is the expansion of the skin creating wrinkles or folds in the lids that convey fatigue or age. If a patient is inquiring about a face-lift, the lids have usually progressed sufficiently in the aging process that a blepharoplasty is an appropriate accompaniment.

The eyelids are delicate, and at the same time, tough. They heal exceedingly rapidly and well, leaving little evidence that they have been altered. They heal so well and are so forgiving that many physicians with little training in aesthetic surgery get out their cookbooks and do unimaginative blepharoplasties and get by with it. The results are often not the best, but the patients are improved and don't know it could be better.

The most common problem the plastic surgeon sees is the patient who has far too much skin in the upper eyelids due to age or the result of one's genetic heritage. This skin can hang beyond the lid margin and interfere significantly with the upward and outward gaze. Lifting the lids up to see can be tiring. We have all seen elderly people with this problem. I often wish it were appropriate to nudge someone at the grocery store and tell him that he would really see better and tire less easily if he would have an upper-lid blepharoplasty. In the severe cases where pictures show the skin pushing the lashes down and visual field tests show limitation of upward gaze, this procedure may be paid for through Medicare (1989).

The upper blepharoplasty for blepharochalasis (this is what it is called) can usually be done in less than 30 minutes, under local anesthesia, and in the most informal of operating settings. I usually don't sedate such patients. Immediately after the procedure they go home with a pain pill (to help them deal with the discomfort that occurs when the anesthetic wears off) and some witch hazel-soaked pads to relieve the itching.

Black eyes follow, but the immediate opening of what has become built-in blinds is gratefully received.

Stitches come out in three or four days and the swelling and bruises around the eyes are usually gone within 12 days. Patients often complain, at first, that they have to wear dark glasses because they haven't seen so much light in years.

Occasionally, some herniated fat is removed during the blepharoplasty along with some extra skin. This takes a little longer and has little other effect except that the eyelids will look better after the operation.

Aesthetic Blepharoplasty.
Unless this procedure is done on someone who has severe blepharochalasis, it is usually not covered by insurance and if it is, only the upper lid surgery will be compensated.

The Problem
Some people, as a part of their design, have more fat in their eyelids than others. In some it is evident in childhood; in others, it becomes evident with age. This can be a reason for a blepharoplasty in a young patient who wants to get rid of the bags in the eyelids.

Aesthetic blepharoplasty is done by first removing a pattern of skin from the lids that the surgeon determines is excess. Often, following this, a strip of the thin muscle that closes the eye is removed from beneath the skin. This depends upon the preoperative condition. Extra fat, known to be present from the preoperative examination, is removed and the skin is closed. A skilled surgeon will vary the amounts of each of these steps, guided by the preoperative condition and his objective.

It is possible, for example, to make a fairly sharp fold in the upper lid where one is absent. This is often done for Asian patients who want to have the upper lid fold, that is often missing, created or made more prominent. This modification is in popular demand in Asia and Hawaii.

Some surgeons feel that everyone should have a definite fold in the upper lid and will incorporate this modification to suit their taste. The sophisticated shopper

45

who has a soft, foldless lid and likes it, should be careful to point this out to the surgeon. The only patients I have ever seen who were really dissatisfied with their blepharoplasty, other than those with complications, are the few who have come in with preoperative pictures saying, "He changed my looks when I didn't ask him to. I only wanted to look younger." The upper lid which previously was soft and foldless now had a well-defined fold. This is called the supratarsal fold. It is difficult to reverse.

The Procedure

Blepharoplasty takes an hour or two. It is usually done under local anesthesia with sedation. The local is put directly into the lids with a fine needle. Some people panic at the idea of surgery about their eyes, so it can be done under general anesthesia. After the local anesthesia, it is painless, though one might feel a tug now and then. You don't see the operation as your eyes are closed, except when the surgeon asks you to open them for a short time. After the operation, some surgeons blindfold their patients for a few hours. I'm not certain why, but it does no harm and may reduce swelling. The lids are a bit painful as the anesthesia wears off. The lids may also ache a little, and they usually itch until the stitches come out in two to four days.

Cool compresses will help relieve the itching. It is O.K. to take a shower. Most people don't wear their contact lenses for a few days, but I know some slip them in quite soon after the operation. Removal is more difficult. If the patient will ask the person who fits the lenses, it is possible to get a suction device that will greatly facilitate getting the contact lenses out. They don't encourage the use of these devices, but can often be talked into providing one for the blepharoplasty patient.

Often a brow-lift, or the part of a face-lift that lifts the side of the eyebrow, will tighten the upper lid significantly. Therefore, it is wise to do these operations first and then work on the upper lids. Experienced surgeons can

46

make these assessments without doing the brow-lift first, but it is safer to keep the order in mind.

Once in a while a patient will come complaining of droopy eyelids who truly has droopy lids as well as excess skin. In these cases there has been some stretching or weakening of the muscle that lifts the upper lid. When this occurs, it is possible to correct the problem (called "dehiscence ptosis") at the same time as the blepharoplasty. Insurance will often cover this.

Complications

Complications of blepharoplasty include the usual hazards of surgery. Bleeding is uniformly shown by black eyes. Bleeding that would interfere with health is almost impossible following a blepharoplasty. However, I once operated on a man whose postoperative bleeding brought the profession's attention to, and his awareness of, a diagnosis of a form of hemophilia. Blood clots in the muscle of the lower lid may hold the lid below its usual position for a few weeks, but this is unusual.

Infection is quite rare in eyelids after surgery, but it has happened. I once saw a woman who thought a fever, redness and pain were to be expected after her eyelid surgery (performed by another surgeon). Her streptococcal infection progressed to the point that she had a very unpleasant result with the loss of some skin. This is the only case that I recall where an infection occurred following a blepharoplasty.

We must mention the rare but significant accompaniment of all eyelid surgery. It is possible that a complication will adversely effect vision. Hemorrhage in the back of the eye is the best known cause, but there are others. I don't know the statistics on this. I suspect no one does, but it is very, very rare. When it occurs, we usually hear about it in medical journals.

Eyelid aesthetic surgery is one of the most rewarding of the procedures in plastic surgery to combat aging. Like the other procedures for aging skin, the operation only sets back the clock which will continue to advance. It takes about seven years for the lids become about the same again. The benefit of this procedure is permanent to the degree that one never looks as bad as he would have at the age he is. It is also probably the easiest procedure for the patient to endure.

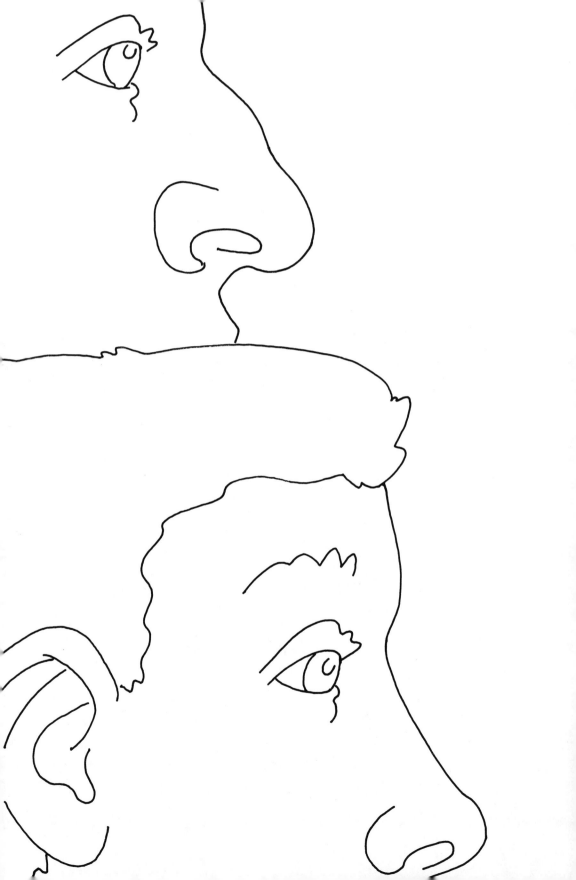

8

For A More
Stylish Nose

The nose is in the center of the face and is more functional than a thing of beauty. Its delicacy can make a cover girl beguiling. Its grossness gives the cowboy and the pugilist the appearance of masculinity. But, when encountering another individual we want to impress, it doesn't supply us with much information about how we're doing; the rest of the face holds these expressive qualities.

The nose is like the dividing line in the middle of a highway. It separates the cars, but we don't remember whether it was white or yellow, dashed or solid. Its importance was only its presence; if it were absent, we would certainly be aware of it, but the action takes place on both sides of it.

Fundamentally, the nose is a roof over the hole in the skull through which a person breathes. Unless the skull is modified for some reason, the nasal reconstruction must fit comfortably on this foundation. For this reason, attempts to reduce a nose too much leaves a result that is conspicuous and almost a deformity. Many such noses can be seen while walking down Fifth Avenue on a sunny afternoon.

An interest in noses is an affliction of plastic surgeons, otorhinolaryngologists, and a section of society which selects itself to be candidates for nasal reformation. The operation is called "rhinoplasty" by the surgeons, "nose job" by the public. It is done for those in society who have identified their nose as a feature they don't enjoy. Those who have a rhinoplasty are almost always disappointed that their friends don't really notice the result. The most the patient can expect is a question about a new hairstyle or new makeup, although those few acquaintances who also have a special interest in noses may notice.

The nose does most of its growing during puberty-- earlier in girls than boys. The nose is usually near adult size 18-months after the first menstrual period, and when the young man begins shaving daily. The nose continues to enlarge throughout life, but very slowly. The growth of the nose at puberty and elongation of the face between the eyes and the mouth are the things that change faces from those of children to those of young adults. We prefer not to do aesthetic surgery on a nose until the patient has passed this growing period.

Rhinoplasty on the right patient is a wonderful operation. It takes away a stigma that seriously degrades the self-image. The problem is that it is very difficult to determine what the benefit will be for a particular patient in the time the plastic surgeon has to spend with any pre-operative patient. Most patients who decide to have something done about their nose and who present themselves for this purpose turn out to be good candidates for surgery, if they continue to decide to have it done after full disclosure of the events, methods and consequences of the surgery.

The most unhappy cosmetic surgical patients I have seen, have been those who had rhinoplasties at the suggestion of a doctor or friend and had not spontaneously decided they wanted something done about their nose. It is easy for a doctor to suggest an operation to some patients, particularly if he wants to do a few. The results are sometimes quite tragic.

Rhinoplasty is a fascinating operation for the surgeon, and is my favorite procedure. It is a three dimensional challenge where the materials one is working with are unpredictable in thickness, elasticity, strength, and potential for resistance to the forces of the ever-present scarring that will follow the procedure. The result is never perfect, but patients tend to like the improvements for which the surgeon is eternally grateful.

Rhinoplasty is an operation where the result is very dependent upon the experience of the surgeon. I tell my residents that they should, when out in private practice, pay the first 50 patients on whom they do rhinoplasties, do the next 50 for free, and then start charging for the operation with a clear conscious. Of course, none of them listen seriously to this, but the sensible ones don't accept difficult noses until they have done a number of those noses large enough that there is margin for error. The most difficult noses are those that are small and need only minor corrections.

Crooked noses are fascinating in many ways. They are the product of disturbed internal and external anatomy. Patients are most aware of them in pictures. We all get used to what we see in the mirror and assume it is the norm. In fact, what we see in the mirror is reversed, and we become used to our face backwards. When we see pictures of ourselves (the way everyone else has gotten used to seeing us), it seems backwards to us. So, if one's nose is deviated to the side by 15 degrees (actually not noticed as crooked by one's friends), one sees it in a picture as 15 degrees to the other side, or actually 30 degrees from what we see in the mirror. In this respect, it really looks crooked!! Patients often bring pictures to show the surgeon how crooked the nose is. Because of this, surgeons have mirrors in their offices that reverse the image to help explain this asymmetry to their patients.

The Operation

The nose is numbed with local anesthetics that have the ability to limit bleeding, even if the patient is put to sleep. Most rhinoplasties are done with the patient under local anesthesia, but there is no reason not to use general anesthesia if the patient wishes. The patient is sedated and the nose is packed gently with cotton moistened with cocaine solution, and local anesthetic is injected into the skin of the nose. This hurts, but not for long. The cotton is removed and the operation begins.

First, incisions are made inside the nostrils, and using special instruments, the skin is lifted off the skeleton of the nose. If the problem is the typical one where a hump is present and the nose is generally overlarge, the hump is removed and the nasal bones are separated from their attachment to the cheeks. These are then fractured inward to narrow the bridge, thus reducing the upper,

54

bony portion of the nose.

Then, the lower cartilaginous skeleton is reduced and sculpted to allow a new, more delicate and appropriate shape for the nose. This requires the modification of the septum and the two cartilaginous structures that establish the contour of each side of the nose. There are many ways to do this. The surgeon must choose correctly from many options to obtain an acceptable result.

The operation rarely takes more than a couple of hours, often less than an hour when done by a very experienced surgeon. If it is necessary or desirable to do cartilage grafting, bone grafting or other more complex procedures, more time must be spent. There are volumes written for surgeons on the intricate modifications of rhinoplasty, so many in fact, that it is often wiser to know what one should not do rather than to know all the things that one might choose to do to a nose.

It is difficult for the inexperienced, even the unacquainted doctor, to understand how this procedure is done. It has been developed over the last century into an operation requiring unique instruments and unique skills.

The operation is followed by various types of taping of the skin of the nose, followed by a splint secured to the face with adhesive to hold the nose in proper position for healing. Packing the nose is sometimes necessary, though often avoidable--for which a patient should be grateful since the removal of the packing can be the worst part of the procedure. Packing is routinely used if septal surgery is done with the rhinoplasty. Packing is usually removed in a couple of days, and the splint is removed in five to seven days.

When the splint is removed, about 80 percent of the swelling is gone. The rest of the swelling will disappear in another week. There will be some swelling and thickness that will remain for about a year. Socially, no one will notice the changes that occur after three weeks or so, but careful photographic documentation will reveal the changes. The result of a rhinoplasty is usually complete in about two to three weeks.

The typical rhinoplasty patient will carefully inspect the nose soon after the surgery and see that the nose is not perfectly symmetrical. If the patient had similarly inspected the nose prior to surgery, which almost never happens, it would have been obvious that it was not symmetrical in the first place. Faces are never symmetrical and rhinoplasty does not make them so.

Bleeding

Bleeding always follows nasal surgery and patients should not be alarmed by it unless it is excessive. In addition, black eyes almost always occur and are gone in about 10 days. Activities should be limited for about 10 days after a rhinoplasty to keep the blood pressure down and limit bleeding. If a nose bleed occurs, sit down, head above heart, and put a cold wet cloth at the end of the nose. Press gently, do not dab as this will often make the bleeding continue. The nose bleed should stop in a few minutes--if it doesn't, call your doctor.

We now know that aspirin is a common cause of postoperative bleeding and advise our patients to refrain from its use for at least 10 days before surgery. A single aspirin tablet will increase a person's bleeding time for 10 days.

Pain

Immediately after a rhinoplasty it is common to have a significance headache for a couple of hours. When this passes, pain is often not a problem. It may be annoying but not disabling.

Infection

Infection, even after an operation on the nose, is rare. Persistent pain is a symptom of infection and should be reported.

The Septum
The nasal septum is the wall between the nostrils. It is almost always crooked or deviated to some extent. Severe deviations cause obstruction to breathing and contribute to sinusitis. Often when a patient presents a crooked nose for correction, a crooked septum is a part of the problem and must be corrected to straighten the nose. So, the correction of a deviated septum is often done at the same time as a rhinoplasty to improve the appearance of the nose. Frequently, one procedure cannot be done well without the other. Correction of the deviated septum can be done without altering the appearance of the nose in most cases. Correction of a crooked nose cannot be done without correcting the septum.

One of the problems with this procedure is getting insurance companies to cover septal correction along with the rhinoplasty. Frequently, there is a conflict between insurance companies and the patient who has a deviated septum and a desire for a rhinoplasty at the same time. This problem has been compounded by some surgeons who have attempted to help their patients defraud their insurance companies to obtain coverage for cosmetic surgery, making the companies particularly alert.

Sometimes it is desirable to use septal cartilage to build up parts of nose in rhinoplasty, so septal surgery is not always done for nasal obstruction. Similarly, bits of cartilage are occasionally taken from the ear for the same reason.

Secondary Surgery
Every surgeon who does rhinoplasty has an occasional patient who requires a second operation to get the best result. Sometimes things do not break where they should. At other times, it turns out after surgery that too much or too little was removed, and a second operation would make things a bit better. If possible, such revisions should wait about a year after the initial operation so the scar has cured and the correction is in its near permanent state.

Most surgeons look at their rhinoplasties a year after the operation and wish they had done a little more or a little less here or there. These efforts at perfection should not, in my opinion, be reason to seduce a satisfied patient back into the operating room. Most patients are happier with the results of their rhinoplasties than are their surgeons. I hope I will never be entirely satisfied with the results of my surgery, for then I would have quit growing as a surgeon.

Rhinoplasty is a great operation for the patient who wants the change it will establish. Unlike surgery for aging, rhinoplasty changes appearance, it does not restore what was there previously. Some surgeons will show the patient what his profile could be like after surgery, using a video camera and a computer. Remember, this is only what you are likely to look like, it will not be exact. Some surgeons may show before and after pictures of cases he may have done. If he is human, he is not likely to show you his average result, only his best. There is no assurance that you will be one of his best results.

With all these warnings, I think it is safe to say that if you want a rhinoplasty and need a surgeon, be sure he is a trained plastic surgeon--one with experience, who is respected by his colleagues, and that you like.

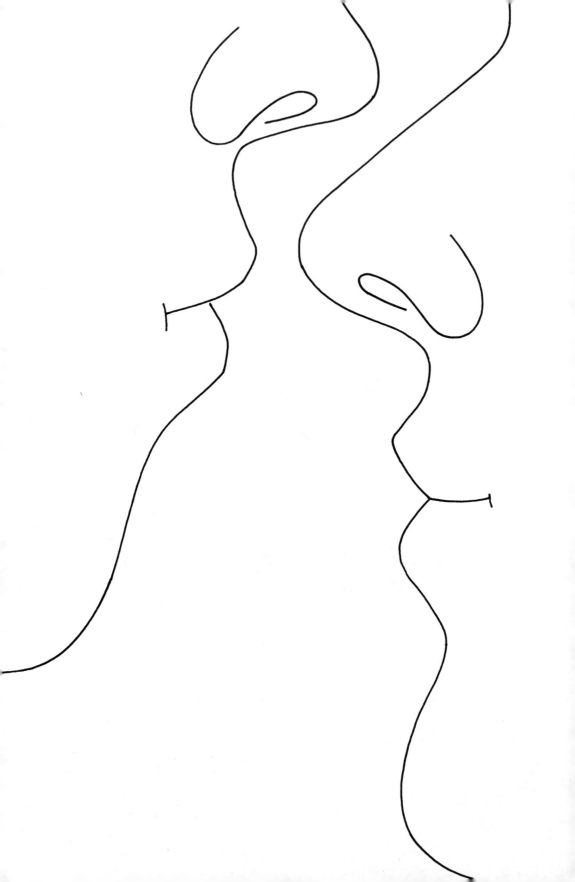

9

I Don't Like
My Chin

Changing the shape of the chin is relatively common in plastic surgery. It is sometimes done as part of the correction of a more severe problem of dental occlusion, or of developmental abnormalities in which the jaw is malformed as a result of a congenital anomaly, or heredity. Very large chins are also a sign of a condition called acromegally that is the result of a tumor of the pituitary gland.

Reconstructive surgical procedures of the jaws are major operations done by plastic and maxillofacial surgeons after considerable rearranging of the teeth by orthodontists. These operations often require extensive carpentry of the mandible and facial skeleton, with frequent bone grafting and fixation of the parts with metal plates and screws that are similar to tiny erector sets. The results are often quite dramatic, both from the standpoint of dental function and appearance. The frequency of these extensive manipulations for purely aesthetic reasons has increased as the profession has gained experience, the necessary equipment to perform the operations has become more refined, and the risks of such surgery have diminished.

The most common manipulations of the chin for aesthetic reasons involve only the front part of the jaw and do not affect the teeth or dental function. There are two definite schools of thought about how the front of the jaw should be manipulated, and this is influenced by the experience of the surgeon and how familiar he is with sculpting the facial bones.

When the chin sticks out too much, there is little to do but to cut some of the front of the jaw (the mandible) off to create a more desirable aesthetic profile. This is usually done through incisions made inside the lower lip with elegant saws powered by tiny turbines, and driven by gas under pressure. These procedures are done, often under local anesthesia, in a setting not unlike a dental office. The results are most gratifying in the properly selected case.

More frequently, the jaw is modified in the opposite direction because it needs more projection. The methods of accomplishing this are placed into two classes. Most commonly, chins are enlarged by adding an implant of silicone, either solid or an encapsulated gel, a material called Proplast (a biologically acceptable porus plastic material), or a variety of other materials, usually plastics, which are being developed for human bone augmentation. Such implants are usually of prefabricated shapes, and a selection is available to the surgeon. Each surgeon has his favorite method of chin implantation and there is not a great deal of difference in the expected result or risk.

The second group of procedures for chin enlargement are methods of modifying the mandible such as cutting off the lower edge, advancing it forward, and securing it there with screws or wires. Sometimes, if the jaw is too long vertically, and too short horizontally, the lower part of the jaw is trimmed off and secured in front of the upper portion to correct both deficiencies. These procedures are usually done by the surgeons who frequently do more major maxillofacial surgery.

I know surgeons who will never use an implant, but will always modify the bone. I also know surgeons who have never modified the bone and have done hundreds of chin implants on patients who are sufficiently satisfied that the surgeon has felt free to continue to use his implants.

The disadvantages of implants are that they will sometimes erode the bone and make a hole in it, into which the implant sinks and causes some loss of projection. It is my opinion that implants erode the bone until they make a surface so close to the opposite of itself that it will no longer move on the bone and erode it. Much is written about this erosion, but it rarely seems to cause any problems for the teeth, the jaw, or the patient. Some newer chin implants are made of materials that appear to leave the bone unmolested.

Chin implants can be placed either through an incision behind the lower lip, or in the skin behind the point of the chin. They rarely become infected, even when put in through the mouth. They are often used in procedures to correct a double-chin in an older patient, and to assist in the reshaping of the neck that slopes low and back from the chin. Some surgeons encourage the use of chin implants to improve the profile of patients on whom they are reducing the size of the nose.

This latter question, chin implants with rhinoplasties, is an almost religious issue. Some surgeons feel the need to encourage patients to have chin implants with their rhinoplasties, and others would never suggest a chin implant to a patient who needs a reduction rhinoplasty. I am in the latter group. One of my dear friends, who has practiced almost as long as I have, has done at least a couple of hundred chin implants on his rhinoplasty patients. I have done, perhaps, three. We can discuss this difference, freely, as we can discuss his Catholicism and my Protestant inclinations. In fact, when I was talking to him this morning in preparation for writing this chapter, we were conjecturing that his attitude was based on the fact that he has a dominant chin, and I have one which does not call attention to itself. We laughed, but I suspect there is some truth in this.

Certainly the sophisticated shopper should look carefully at the recommendation to have a chin implant at the time of rhinoplasty. It is easy to do a chin implant on a separate occasion. I don't recall a patient with whom I discussed a chin implant as a possible event after a reduction rhinoplasty who came in to have one. Although there is one exception I will never forget who insisted that I should have done a chin implant. I did it in a second operation, and two days later she insisted I take it out.

One way to see if you want to have a chin implant is to ask your surgeon to inject a few cubic centimeters, or less, of local anesthesia into the front of your chin. Look quickly, or even take a picture, and you can see roughly what an implant will do.

Orthodontists who live their lives looking at teeth

and profiles, often recommend chin implants or chin modifications. They may, in our culture, be the cause of more such operations than would ever occur without their aesthetic recommendations. In my years of practice, chin augmentation is one of the least frequent reasons patients come to see me, but those who express concern, and are operated upon, are some of my most grateful patients.

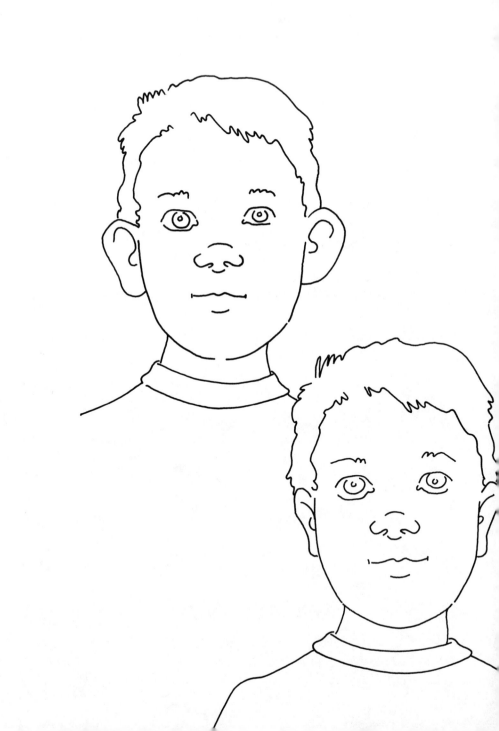

10

But My Ears
Stick Out

The ear of a man is noticed if it is absent, has a bite out of it, or sticks out too far. Otherwise it has little significance.

It is not our purpose to talk about deformed or absent ears, what we will discuss are prominent ears. Prominent ears are embarrassing. Grandmothers try to hold them back unsuccessfully with tape or caps. Ultimately, either they part the girl's hair too much or they stick out too far on the thin boy's head, and we see them in consultation. If the boys will wait until puberty when their shoulders grow out from their necks, the ears won't appear so prominent.

At least 80 percent of the growth of the ear is completed by the age of six, so we prefer to wait until then to operate. It is also easier to deal with a child who wants his ears fixed, than with one whose parents want the ears fixed. A child who wants the operation is willing to put up with the inconvenience and discomfort with understanding. Additionally, I think a bit of teasing helps develop a useful level of compassion for other's afflictions.

In the 50s and early 60s, short hair cuts were the style and otoplasty was relatively common. In the 70s and early 80s, the long hair styles hid many prominent ears. Now, short haircuts are bringing business to plastic surgeons.

The correction of prominent ears appears easy when done with skill. It requires great intellectual flexibility on the part of the surgeon. No two ears are alike even on the same person and usually, slightly different operations are done on each side.

In most cases the operation can be done with a local anesthetic. The ear is thin and can be quickly made exceedingly numb. The procedure doesn't take much more than an hour for both ears. The patient's face need not be covered as he can't see the operation, he can only hear it. The environment can be made light, pleasant, musical and conversational, so that once the annoyance of the local anesthesia is completed, the operation can be much like a game for the patient, who is usually a child.

We normally take a strip of skin off the back of the ear and then carve, thin, bend, suture, and/or remove part of the cartilage to achieve the desired result. Slight bleeding is controlled, and the wound in the back of the ear is closed with sutures that won't need to be taken out. A rather bulky, protective dressing follows which is left on for a few days, longer in children than adults.

Postoperative pain is often severe for a few hours, particularly in adults. Children often don't notice it. I generally don't premedicate children much for this surgery as they are unaccustomed to altered states of consciousness and do better when they are intellectually intact. Instead, I give them something for pain at the end of the operation when they might need it. Adults always require pain medications, but four to five hours after the operation most patients of any age have little pain unless they are bumped. The ears appear bruised for a couple of weeks and are tender for a few more.

Complications in this procedure are exceedingly rare. They include, as in all surgery, bleeding, infection, adverse scarring, and a poor result.

The results are rarely perfect. The operated ear would rarely pass inspection by a plastic surgeon looking for evidence that an operation had been done. But, the patient and his mother are usually quite pleased, as there are few ear inspectors in our culture.

This is a fairly common operation. It's been done on one of our more recent presidents, a number of movie stars, some members of royal families, and I'll bet you've never noticed.

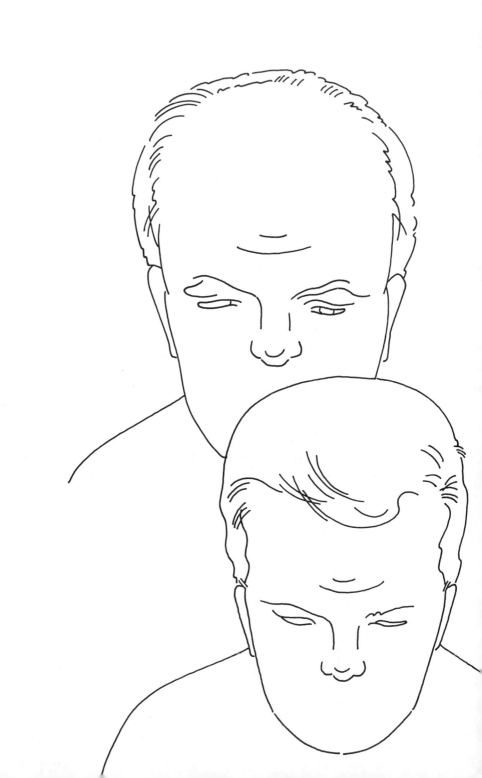

11

I'm Losing My Hair And I Don't Like Wigs

About 60 percent of the male population of the United States will ultimately become bald to some extent. None of these men like it. Some live with their baldness; others, annoyed or depressed by it, will do something. Some are talked into it by their wives, but most seek help on their own.

Baldness is inherited. In fact, most things about hair is hereditary. Coarseness, durability, quantity, distribution, color, and the tendency toward graying are all evidences of our membership in a particular race, nationality, and family.

Baldness can be prevented by castration. It does not occur in men who are hypogonadal and who have low levels of testosterone, the principal male hormone. The fact that baldness is a sign of virility is not very encouraging to the men who simply don't like the loss of their hair. One of my anatomy professors, who was quite bald, used to amuse us with the pun, "Eunuchs are never bald."

There is an increasing willingness on the part of aging men in our culture to do something about the evidence of age our hair expresses. Many middle-aged men are dying their hair. Others buy wigs or seek medical attention. Herb Caen, a San Francisco columnist, recently described a wealthy San Francisco businessman who had a collection of almost identical wigs, each with longer hair than the preceding one, so that it would look like his hair was growing between haircuts.

During my lifetime, the quality of wigs has improved greatly, and the methods of their application and attachment has also improved. One of my younger colleagues is wearing a small "patch wig" in his central bald spot which is really quite excellent and only detectable when he leans over.

Some wigs are held on by attaching them to stitches through the scalp, but most are fastened with constantly improving adhesives which are causing less and less dermatitis. Dermatologists still see wig wearers with scalp irritation, but those instances are becoming less frequent.

Surgical approaches to baldness were rare events, usually done for baldness after injury or burns until 1959, when Norman Orentreich, a New York dermatologist, reported his success with grafting clusters of hair follicles in small round pieces of scalp (taken from the hairy sides of the scalp) and placed in the bald areas. These punch grafts were quite successful and his discovery has created a sub-profession of doctors who do little else but care for male pattern baldness.

The technique has been perfected through experience. Free grafts of skin bearing hair are now used (sometimes in square, rather than round pieces and occasionally, in strips). Smaller grafts are used to allow feathering at the edges of the grafted area at the top of the forehead.

Everything has its disadvantages. Hair grows normally, generally over an area. The grafts are, of necessity, in clusters. This can be seen on close inspection by those who chance to look for it. Before the process was refined, the grafts were so regularly placed they looked like tiny rice paddies. Now, they are placed more at random, so it isn't as likely that an observer will look down the rows as if looking at an orchard.

Scalp reduction, or the partial removal of the bald section, is becoming more popular and reduces the area of the problem significantly. A newer approach is to expand the hair bearing scalp using silicone balloons or expanders which are surgically placed below the desired area. These balloons can be inflated by injection into a special device through the skin until the hair bearing scalp is enlarged to allow greater areas of baldness to be removed.

Procedure

Almost all surgery for the treatment of baldness is done in ambulatory settings under local anesthesia. Sometimes the grafting procedures are done on consecutive days. The amount of social or occupational disability depends on the patient's attitude and situation. Most patients can get back to their usual routine with some creative hair dressing in less than a week. Pain is usually not severe after the procedure, but the first couple of days may be uncomfortable.

Other surgical approaches for balding include taking large flaps of scalp from the hairy sides of the head and moving them across the front of the bald area to establish a hairline above the forehead. The scalp has excellent blood supply, so that strips of hair bearing scalp over an inch wide can be five times as long as the width. This strip of skin is lifted from the back forward, and the donor area closed. Another incision is made, typically where the hairline should be; and after removing some of the bald scalp, the flap is turned at a right angle and stitched into the new position. There are many patterns of flaps available for this type of hair transfer. The edges of the flaps are commonly obscured by the use of punch grafts to feather the conspicuous edges.

Complications
Some follicles are damaged in the move and the result is that the hair that grows may be different in texture and somewhat curlier, which can be difficult to manage and somewhat annoying. Some grafts will tend to hump up a bit, and this irregularity may be noticeable. There are techniques to improve this. The scars of the donor site cannot be hidden from the barber who usually knows what has happened anyway. There is always a clue to the interested observer. Nonetheless, most hair transplants done by pros are sufficiently good that normal observers won't notice them in social contact. Many hair transplant patients wear bifocals and it is difficult to see one's scalp in detail through the part of the lens required to see things sharply up close.

ஃ

The methods of hair transplantation and movement, designed for the treatment of baldness, have many applications in the care of hairless scalps from injury or burns. Occasionally, women have patterns of baldness that require such treatment as well.

As you can see, the surgical treatment of baldness is becoming quite an art. There are many techniques, and, as is present in most surgical fields, there is a relationship between the likelihood of a good result and the experience of the surgeon. So the sophisticated shopper should feel free to ask the surgeon about his favorite methods and his experience.

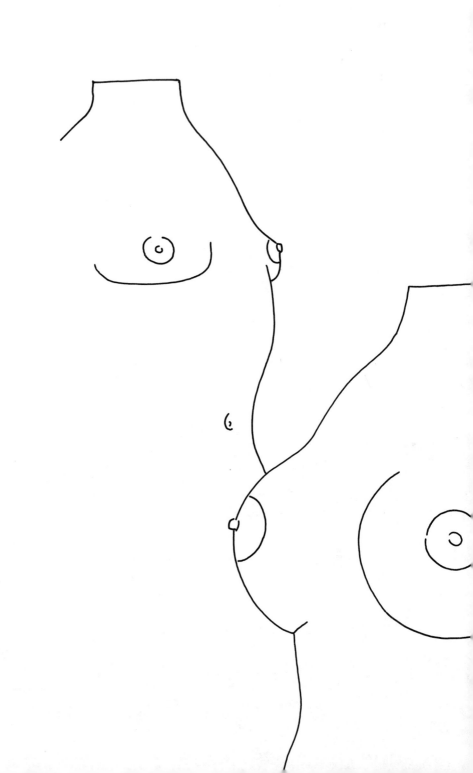

12

I Must Have
Larger Breasts

Breast augmentation doesn't make sense to much of the medical profession and much of the public. But for women who see their small breasts as a problem, this procedure is a revelation. The results are good enough that as many as 85 percent of women who have the surgery are sufficiently satisfied, that they don't return to the surgeon for follow-up visits after a short time. They accept the new contour as their own and often don't think very much about it.

This operation simply involves making a space beneath the breast and filling it with a substance felt to be safe and tolerable by the surgeon.

Silicone comes in many forms, liquid to handball rubber hard. It is used in many medical and commercial applications. A couple of decades ago it was popular in parts of the world to inject breasts with liquid silicone; but became unpopular when it formed lumps that could be mistaken for cancer. It also diffused into the skin making funny spots and ulcerations. At this point, the FDA put limits on its use in the U.S. which has, like most bureaucratic regulations, been only partially effective.

Historically, the first breast augmentations were done with carved polyvinyl (kitchen) sponges. Unfortunately, it turned out that these sponges developed bone in their pores after a few years. Then came silicone rubber and silicone gel developed by Dow Corning Corporation and tested by two surgeons in Texas. Silicone became the standard material for breast implants as a result.

Now, silicone implants are usually breast-shaped bags of clear silicone rubber filled with either saline solution, or more commonly, silicone gel. Some implants have double lumens with an inner shell containing silicone gel, and an outer one containing saline solution. Some have the silicone outside.

Saline-filled silicone implants are the safest implants to have because if they break, (and they do) only salt water leaks into the surrounding tissues which is quickly absorbed and excreted. When a silicone gel-filled implant breaks, the gel is quite reactive and causes various unpleasant, but usually fairly harmless, foreign body reactions. These may manifest as lumps in the breast implant capsule. The gel is rarely pushed away from the implant capsule which can cause complications.

Controversies In Breast Implantation

It has been recently reported that some studies conducted by Dow Corning Corp. have revealed that silicone in rats is associated with a form of cancer called fibrosarcoma. The news reports suggested that Dow and the FDA were withholding this information from the public and the medical profession. This resulted in charges and counter charges. It has been known for at least 30 years that fibrosarcoma occurs in rats in the presence of smooth foreign bodies such as glass, metal and plastics. It does not occur in the presence, for example, of fabrics made of the same plastics that induce the tumor in smooth form. There are literally millions of foreign bodies of the types that cause cancer in rats present in the tissues of living people. Shell fragments and bullets from wars, pieces of glass from accidents, orthopedic surgical implants, screws and plates, and plastic and metal plates in skulls are a few of the more common examples. There has been no reported fibrosarcoma in association with a human breast implant or any other silicone implant. So, it would appear that this is much ado about nothing.

There have been, of course, breast cancers, in patients who have had implants. There should be as there are over two million breast implants in the American population. Breast cancer does not occur more frequently in women with breast implants. There is, in fact, a research study in which a group of patients who had implants had less breast cancer than a comparable group of women. This is not well understood. There is only conjecture that women with smaller breasts may have less breast cancer; no one has studied this.

Two issues that are getting press about breast implants should be mentioned:

First, it is said that mammograms are not as effective in patients who have had breast implants. It is probably true that, if no consideration is given to the fact that there is an implant present, mammograms will not be as effective. If, however, the study is done the way it should be in the implanted breast, it is possible that it will be even more effective, as the radiologist will be looking more carefully. There is a significant difference in quality of mammograms from laboratory to laboratory even without the added consideration of implants.

Second, there is a study which shows that a group of women who have had breast cancer after having implants, have come to the doctor when the tumor was more advanced than a similar group who have not had breast implants. This is likely to have nothing to do with the implants, but a great deal to do with the people who have the operation. Women frequently will watch a breast lump for too long, in the hope that it will go away before they go to the doctor. Such denial would certainly be more prevalent in women whose concern about their breasts brought them to a plastic surgeon in the first place.

The Procedure
The operation is usually done as an outpatient procedure. It takes less than an hour and a half to do both sides. Either a local or general anesthetic can be used. Pain is usually not severe after surgery. I advise my patients to take a couple of days off from strenuous work. In a couple of weeks, recovery is usually complete, except for a little tenderness and some swelling.

It is wise to wear a bra at all times for the first couple of weeks. If the family has a tendency toward droopy breasts before implantation, it is better not to go braless for extended periods as the implants have sufficient weight to stretch the skin. (The implants weigh about the same as an equal amount of breast tissue.)

Incisions on the breast are usually quite inconspicuous. The most common are made along the lower part of the breast where the marks of the bra usually show. They are usually about two inches long. The second most common incision is made around the lower part of the areola. Less common are incisions in the armpits or across the center of the areola. Since the normal patient has a life expectancy much longer than our experience with any implant, I assume that the implants will, for some reason, need to be replaced in the future. For this reason, I prefer the incision under the breast which passes immediately behind the breast without going through it. This is less likely to cause nipple numbness, less hemorrhage, and infection even though these complications are rare.

The implant can be placed under the breast or under the pectoral muscle. The choice is up to the surgeon and patient. There are good arguments for both. Some feel there is less encapsulation with submuscular implants. In addition, there is distortion of the breasts with arm movement. The implant can also be less palpable if it is under the muscle. The most common argument for submuscular placement is that it reduces the frequency of hardness and encapsulation, but many surgeons are not convinced that this is true.

Any choice has some disadvantage. There are implants with only saline inside them, implants with only silicone gel, implants with one chamber inside the other, gel in one and saline in the other, implants with smooth surfaces, implants with rough surfaces, implants with polyurethane foam bonded to the surface (said to disrupt the direction of the scar fibers so there is less contracture, hardness), and implants that have devices that allow salt water to be injected into them through the skin so the size can be changed. These are called "expanders", and are used to stretch the skin slowly to accommodate a larger implant, usually after breast cancer surgery where implants are used for breast reconstruction. Expanders of this sort are used extensively in many types of reconstructive surgery, wherever skin can be stretched to make more available.

Complications

Serious complications of breast augmentation do occur, but they are quite rare. The most likely complications are encapsulation or implant failure; both are likely to require second operations.

The most annoying problem after surgery is encapsulation which makes the breast firm. It is the result of shrinking of the fibrous capsule the body forms around the implant. It is easy to describe, but very difficult to explain. It is said to be due to many different things, and it is possible that all of the explanations are, in part, correct. Some of the possible causes are bacterial contamination, hemorrhage or bruising, leakage of silicone gel or microfragmentation of silicone, or a genetic tendency to scar.

Surgeons have different methods to deal with the resulting hardness. Some insist that the patient push the implants around in the breast several times a day to keep the capsule larger than the implant, others tell their patients not to bother. Sometimes, the surgeon will compress the implant to break the capsule, which makes it softer. This is not comfortable, and if effective, should probably be done repeatedly as the capsule recontracts. This method is safer with saline implants because if the implant breaks only salt water is pushed out into the breast tissue.

⁊ꙮ

Every surgeon has his favorite method of breast augmentation and can justify his choice convincingly. None is probably entirely right and none, entirely wrong. The choice of a breast augmentation surgeon is difficult, but since there are many experienced plastic surgeons, it is not a decision like choosing a heart surgeon. Most gynecologists or general practitioners have seen many patients who have had breast augmentations and heard how they feel about their surgeons. Such doctors are a valuable source of referral.

The most uniform thing one can say about patients who have had breast augmentation is that they utterly refuse to have the implants removed permanently for any cause. This is certainly an indication of satisfaction that results from this procedure.

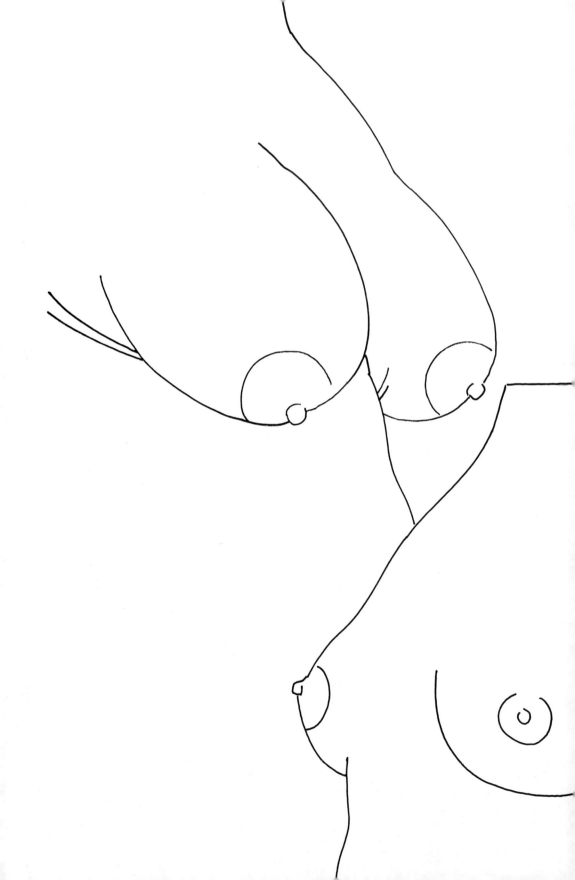

13

For A
Smaller Breast

We learned about breasts in the National Geographic. We saw that they varied in size and shape. We saw thin breasts that fell to the knees. Large globular breasts that looked like a backpack worn backwards. Small elegant breasts such as forgotten sculptors memorialized in Grecian marble. Then came Marilyn Monroe who was, for her time, the model to which the American middle class should aspire. She was a C-plus or D-minus cup size and was the model for her time in history.

Times have now changed and they will again. Breasts were decorative and nonfunctional in the 1950s and 1960s. New mothers who wanted to nurse their babies were strange, and discouraged from this antiquated process. In the late 1980s, nursing is the thing to do. Researchers have found it enhances immunities and builds a bond between mother and child. It also keeps dad from having to get up. It is a rite of the mother and child.

Breasts are secondary sex organs. They participate heavily, or lightly, in a woman's self-image. If they are too large or too droopy, and the husband agrees, the woman may come to the plastic surgeon for relief. The reduction or reshaping of breasts can be both functional and cosmetic. It is always cosmetic in the sense that the shape is better if the operation works.

Function depends upon how much agony is caused by heavy breasts pulling down on the shoulders, creating grooves where the bra straps cut into the skin. Tenderness results from the tourniquet effect of the brassiere holding the breast in. Backache results from the postural stress. The largest breast I have participated in reducing was 10 pounds on each side. In Tanzania, I once saw a 12-year old girl in the hospital who had breasts weighing 55 pounds each, lying in bed beside her.

Researchers have found no correlation between breast size and breast cancer. It is interesting, though, that a study series, conducted on women in Los Angeles who had breast-augmentation, found the frequency of cancer less than that of an age-matched group of women. This single study may suggest that smaller breasts have less cancer.

Breast size is hereditary as are most things related to our appearance. There is also a condition called virginal hypertrophy of the breasts in which girls develop very large, melon-like breasts at puberty. These girls have no particular hormonal disturbance, only breasts that grow too large, too rapidly. In our breast-oriented culture, they suffer greatly from the comments of their peers and are, perhaps, the most grateful for breast reduction.

Husbands have a great deal to do with whether breast reductions get done. I recall a 74-year old women who had large, pendulous breasts, and who, within hours of having buried her husband, came to my office requesting a breast-reduction. She told me he had forbidden her to have such surgery and she was going to do it now, and she could afford it because he had left her the money.

The Procedure

There are many styles of breast reduction operations. The most common method is one which leaves a scar around the areola (the darker skin around the nipple). Another scar descends from the areola to the fold of skin beneath the breast and another extends from the sternum (near the middle of the chest) to the side of the breast under the armpit in the fold between the lower breast and the chest wall. These scars join in a pattern similar to an anchor. Another, less common method, is one which leaves a scar around the areola with two extensions from the areola to the two ends of the fold beneath the breast. One goes to the sternum, and the other, to the side of the chest; both are on the breast. There are many variations on these two themes.

It is best to talk with your surgeon about what he plans to do. Ask to see pictures of his results--preferably pictures of his results after five years. There is much difference between the immediate result of a reduction mammoplasty, and the result after five years.

When the breasts are very large, it is often desirable

to remove the nipples and place them as a graft on the mound the surgeon creates during the operation. This is particularly applicable in long thin breasts or those where it is necessary to remove more than a pound and a half (think of butter!) of tissue on each side. Otherwise, the nipple is supported on the remaining portion of the breast which provides circulation to keep the nipple alive. In either event, it is likely that sensation of the nipple will be lost. Occasionally, when the nipple is moved on a piece of breast tissue, not grafted, sensation will stay intact, but even then it is usually reduced. Nipple sensation is usually reduced in very large breasts, anyway.

Reduction mammoplasty operations take about two hours. They are usually done under a general anesthetic. Frequently, the patient stays a night in the hospital. In young, healthy women with smaller reductions, surgery is done on an outpatient basis.

The postoperative course is not particularly limiting. The breasts are supported in dressings or special bras for about 10 days. Drains may be used which come out in a day or two. Activities are minimally limited. The discomfort is such that some patients go back to work before the stitches are taken out in five to 10 days. It is often easier to work during the mild postoperative annoyances than it is to stay home. If the nipple is grafted, more attention to the dressing is necessary and office care is a bit more prolonged.

Some breast reduction procedures are done solely for correction of drooping breasts. These are called mastopexy. This involves the removal of skin and reshaping the natural brassiere the skin provides. Women who need mastopexy are those who have skin that has stretched too much. In this procedure, it is common that the peculiarities of the skin will remain and the ultimate result will not be lasting. This is particularly true if the thin skin around the nipple is placed under the breast to support the remaining breast tissue. This skin is designed to stretch with pregnancy, and it will do so if it is placed where it must support the breast against gravity. Some surgeons perform a submuscular breast augmentation at the same time. The muscle then holds up the mass of the breast and will not allow it to become distorted as a result of the weight on the skin flaps.

The amount of breast reduction to be done will influence the design of the operation. This should also be a part of the preoperative discussion. If a small amount of tissue is to be removed, scarring will be less evident after the operation.

Occasionally, undetected breast cancer is removed along with the extra breast tissue. This can be an unpleasant surprise. Subsequent treatment will depend upon the microscopic diagnosis of the tumor, and the result of discussion between the patient and surgeon. Breast reduction or mastopexy is also a part of breast reconstruction after mastectomy, where the opposite breast is reformed to match the reconstructed one.

Scarring after breast reduction is the result of the patient's choice of parents rather than the patient's choice of surgeons or the surgeon's method of wound closure. Scars are quite conspicuous for the first few months after the operation and will very likely spread. A year or two after the surgery, they will fade and become approximately the same color as the breast skin.

Complications

Infection is rare after breast reduction. Bleeding postoperatively is also rare, but once, I had to take a patient back into the operating room to control bleeding. Black and blue bruising is common. Healing difficulties are not uncommon as the wounds are closed under some tension to achieve the desired result. This, if it occurs, will cause postoperative annoyance and make the scars wider and sometimes require minor scar revisions.

A rare and very frustrating complication of breast reduction is the loss of the areola and nipple. It is not uncommon for the early postoperative color of these structures to be odd. Occasionally, as result of blood clotting in the feeding vessels or other causes, the nipple and areola will not survive the transfer to the new breast mound. As a result, the surgeon will need to reconstruct the areola and nipple. The nipple won't be as good as new, but patients usually find them acceptable.

Most patients find the pain after surgery tolerable. Severe postoperative pain is usually related to muscle or internal organs, neither of which are involved in reduction mammoplasty.

ॐ

Breast reduction is a great operation, but it isn't perfect. The results are rarely symmetrical. The scars are evident when you walk out of the shower. The patient forgets the annoyance of large breasts and, typically, after a couple of years, wishes it had come out better. But, it is worthwhile and by far, most patients are glad they had it done.

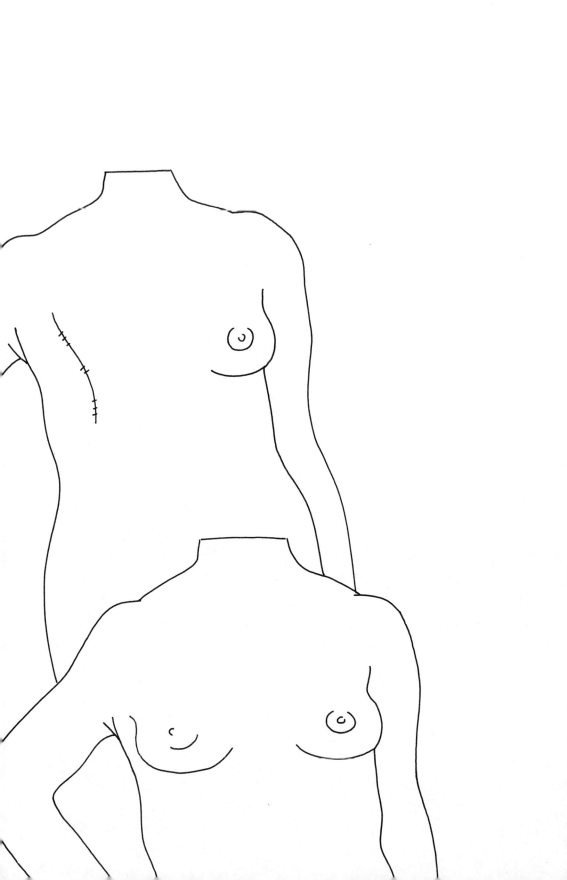

14

I Lost
My Breast

If there is more than one way to treat a condition, then, none is correct. This is an oft repeated statement in medical education.

There are no standard philosophies about breast reconstruction after mastectomy. This is a serious problem. Nine percent of women will eventually have breast cancer. There is not even an accepted standard treatment for breast cancer. The patient sees a doctor, has a biopsy, and then the mystery begins. Shall it be a lumpectomy with radiation, mastectomy, or chemotherapy? There is no doubt that treatment is better than leaving the cancer alone, but no one knows what will ultimately be best. Doctors don't agree. Patients are expected to be "informed", and to participate in the decision. All opinions are biased, so which one should she select?

The first question is, "Do I want my breasts reconstructed?" Some cancer surgeons think reconstruction is inappropriate and advise patients against it. They usually win the first argument. Many surgeons suggest consultation with a plastic surgeon when the diagnosis of breast cancer is a likelihood, or after the biopsy which confirms it. Some patients want the reconstruction started at the time of their breast removal. This is quite possible using a variety of methods such as implants, tissue expanders, moving abdominal skin and shaping it into a "breast", or free transfer of buttock or abdominal skin to make a breast using microscopic connections of arteries and veins to keep the flap of skin alive in the new position.

Other surgeons prefer to wait until the wounds of the breast removal have healed, arguing that the skin, which had previously received much of its circulation from the breast, has had a chance to get used to the reduction of the blood supply and is therefore, more plastic.

The medical profession is divided into enthusiasts for early breast reconstruction, and those who are concerned the patient won't be making her best decision about breast reconstruction when she is in the turmoil of a recent cancer diagnosis. I recall, in the days before immediate reconstruction was commonly accepted, women who were certain that they would have a reconstruction, and who did not, after the fact. I also recall women who were sure they wouldn't, who did. There are also women who have had a mastectomy some time in the past who say, when asked if they have thought about it, "I wouldn't waste my time." Others, who have been off balance for years come in and say, "I'm tired of this, what can you do about it?"

Some enthusiasts believe that the patient is better off if she never has to experience a flat chest. They say she will adapt better to her new life and the shock of now knowing what might be the bottom line. We all know we will die sometime, but we prefer to be ignorant of the cause.

Reconstruction after mastectomy for cancer has been around for about 50 years, but it only became common about 15 years ago. The methods are tremendously varied and none has gained uniform popularity. The sophisticated shopper would be wise to visit at least two plastic surgeons, as we all have pretty fixed ideas and they differ. They are often based, unfortunately, on limited personal experience, or an attempt to improve a particular method without a universal view of what is going on in the field. It is, of course, often better to stay with a surgeon who has a significant experience with one of the methods, and has good results, rather than with one who keeps trying new techniques and never perfects any of them.

The Procedure
Breast reconstruction after mastectomy has three phases. First, the absent breast is replaced by a mound which makes the necessity of wearing a prosthesis in a brassiere unnecessary. Second, a nipple is fabricated from the skin on the face of the mound if the patient wants it. Third, the opposite breast is reshaped and often reduced to resemble the reconstructed side, and to achieve symmetry. Where the breast cancer has a great chance of being

present on the opposite side, the other breast is removed and reconstructed as well. Modification of the opposite breast is often done at the patient's request.

Those of you who have read the preceding two chapters have an idea of the origins of breast reconstruction. The techniques available for breast reconstruction have evolved from the techniques of breast augmentation and reduction with the addition of myocutaneous (muscle-skin) flaps, skin expanders, and microvascular surgery.

Skin expanders are balloons of various sizes made of silicone rubber that have fancy filling valves which can be reached by a needle through the skin. The valve is used to gradually increase the size of the balloon, so the overlying tissues can be stretched to close a nearby wound, or to allow a larger mass to be placed beneath it. The relatively tight skin that follows a mastectomy is often stretched by this means to allow the placement of a breast implant that couldn't be accommodated without the expansion.

The placement of a partially filled expander at the time of a mastectomy is the first step in many breast reconstructions. These are typically replaced by a permanent implant during a second operation when the expansion is completed.

Breast implants of many varieties are used. They are sometimes placed above the pectoral muscle, sometimes below it. For small women, some are placed beneath the muscle at the time of mastectomy. Some implants are smooth on the surface; others are rough and coated with polyurethane foam which many surgeons believe will reduce the occurrence of hardness from implant encapsulation. (This is the formation of a stiff fibrous capsule that captures the implant and makes it hard.)

When it is necessary to add skin to the area, either to increase the space for an implant, or to make a breast of the patient's skin and fat, various skin and fat, or skin, fat and muscle flaps are used to augment the tissues. Flaps can be made from the abdominal wall. This involves moving areas of skin and fat from the adjacent abdomen to the breast area. There are also flaps made of muscle with the overlying skin brought from the back to the breast area.

To bring in sufficient tissue to make a breast without an implant, a large part of the abdominal wall is used. The abdomen is closed as in a tummy tuck and a breast is made of the abdominal muscle, fat and skin. Another procedure brings abdominal skin and fat, or buttock skin and fat, up to the breast, completely detaching it and connecting its arteries and veins to new vessels in the breast area.

Nipple reconstruction is also handled in various ways. If the patient has a large nipple and areola on the intact breast, the nipple can be halved and used as a graft on the needy side. The areola can be halved and grafted as well using a spiral pattern. Nipples have been made of parts of earlobes, parts of the labia, tips of toes, and more recently, usually by making complex pattern of skin flaps and sewing them together to make a nipple. (This is reminiscent of folding paper in Japanese origami.)

The areola is usually made with a skin graft which, if taken from near the pubic hair, will be a darker color, and, it will usually have an irregular surface like an areola. Sometimes bits of ear cartilage or cartilage grafts from tissue banks are slipped beneath the graft to make it irregular Recently, it has become popular to tattoo the nipple and areola in order to gain the proper color. This is done either by the surgeon or a tattoo artist who has been engaged by the surgeon.

The opposite breast may be augmented, reduced, reshaped, or sometimes, removed and reconstructed when the cancer is expected to be bilateral. I have also been asked to remove the other breast by women in order to reduce their fear of cancer.

Radiation treatment of the chest wall makes some additional concerns for the surgeon and the patient undergoing breast reconstruction. After radiation, tissues do not heal as well. This means the approaches and selections of the surgeon must be very conservative. It does not mean reconstruction cannot occur. It is better not to do reconstruction while chemotherapy is going on, but many breast reconstructions have been successful after chemotherapy.

It is common for surgeons to expect patients who embark on breast reconstruction to follow through to the end and have everything done to complete the procedure to the surgeon's satisfaction. Instead, I would advise the patient to regard reconstruction as an a la carte menu. Each stage of the procedure can be considered separately. Often patients are satisfied with the first stage only and don't bother to have a nipple reconstruction. Sometimes they are satisfied without having the opposite breast remodeled. Occasionally, they think they are going to go through the complete reconstruction and instead, stop. Or, they think they will stop at some point and will proceed to completion (sometimes with years between the stages). It is an unpredictable matter of self-perception and personal choice. No course is right or wrong.

As you can see, there are many options in breast reconstruction. Each has it own risk/benefit ratio. Each has its own supporters. Each surgeon has his preference. So, the sophisticated shopper who wants breast reconstruction should be sure she agrees with the surgeon's choice among the alternatives, and, more importantly, she should feel comfortable dealing with the surgeon as she is likely to get to know him well.

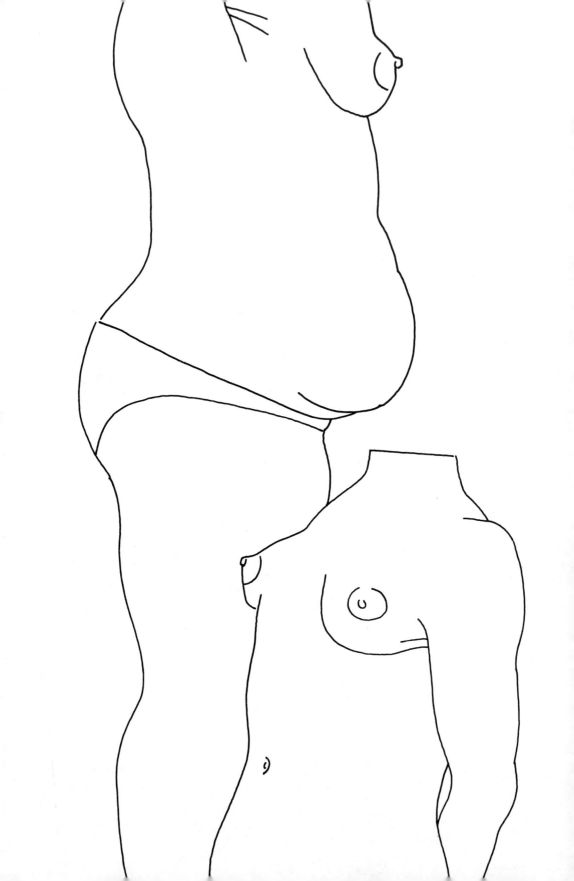

15

The Unsightly Tummy

Called abdominoplasty by surgeons, it is best known as the "tummy tuck" to the general public. This is a category of ways to operate on the lower front of the body to improve the results of genetic selection, overeating, or pregnancy. As always, the way our tummies respond to the stresses of life is determined by our choice of parents.

One of the reasons we look as we do, in both face and body, is the genetically determined way that we deposit fat--where we bank the excess deposits. Such deposits are found in the thighs, breasts, arms, inside the abdomen, under the skin of the abdomen, cheeks, neck, back of the shoulders, buttocks, love handles at the sides of the abdomen, and the Jodhpur deposits on the sides of the thighs.

Similarly, laxity of the skin is a result of parent selection. Abdominoplasty is for people who tend to deposit fat under abdominal skin and for those whose abdominal skin does not shrink back desirably after pregnancy or weight loss. The excess is most noticeable between the navel and the pubic hair.

Abdominoplasty is customarily done under a general anesthetic. It usually take less than two hours to do. It can be done as an outpatient procedure, but most surgeons prefer to hospitalize their patients at least for one night.

Abdominoplasty is a major operation and more involved than other aesthetic surgery. It is often accompanied by muscle tightening procedures performed on the abdominal wall. Typically, this involves bringing the two vertical central muscles of the abdominal wall (the rectus muscles) closer together with heavy sutures.

The abdominoplasty, done on people who have experienced a large weight-loss is often simply the removal of a large wedge of skin and fat from the lower abdomen. The incisions going from one side of the body to the other crossing the lower abdomen. The navel may be removed along with the excess skin.

For the young woman who does not like her wrinkled, puffy lower abdomen, a more acceptable and more complex surgical design is necessary, so that the scars can be hidden under a scanty swimming suit. Here, the incision crosses the top of the pubic hair, and extends out beyond the prominence of the front of the hip bone. The patient may want to choose where this scar goes at the sides because there is no position for the scar that won't show in one style of swimwear or another. We try to put the scars where they will be least visible with the clothing the patient wishes to wear.

Using this lower abdominal incision, the entire skin of the abdomen is separated from the muscle. The umbilicus is left where it belongs by cutting a circle around it. The abdominal skin can then be stretched uniformly downward, the excess is removed and the long wound is closed. A small hole is then cut in the right place to position the belly button. It is then pulled out from under the skin flap and sutured in place. Sometimes it is necessary to have a vertical scar in the lower abdomen. Your surgeon will discuss this with you.

The operation may vary from the standard for a number of reasons--the location of old scars, where the fat or skin may be, or patient preference. The postoperative expectations, which are almost uniform, include some numbness of the skin which improves with time, a fairly conspicuous scar which will fade but not disappear entirely, and some early tenderness which usually goes away. After the operation, it is usually necessary to go about tilted forward at the hips for a few days until the skin and the wound get used to the new tension. It is also not uncommon for the upward pull on the pubic tissues to cause the urinary stream to go forward instead of down for a time, which can be distracting.

Drains, usually suction drains, are often used. These are plastic tubes passed into the wound which suck out any fluid or blood that may accumulate after the surgery. They are a bit of a nuisance, but not particularly uncomfortable. At the end of the tube is a plastic device that applies negative pressure to pull out the drainage. These need to be emptied periodically. The drains are removed when there is little drainage. Some patients need to wear the drains for several days. The device can be hidden under clothing.

Complications

Complications include the usual hazards of surgery: for example, infection, bleeding, poor healing, disappointment with the quality of the result or the effect of the surgery on one's life-style. Most surgeons have heard of, or have seen, the rare situation where, some skin does not survive the procedure and must be removed and a skin graft applied. This may result from infection, tension on the wound, poor blood supply, or bleeding. This complication is quite rare. Another very rare occurrence is the patient who develops a blood clot in a leg which can break off and cause pulmonary emboli (blood clots in the vessels in the lungs). A few of these have been fatal. This problem is a rare complication of all abdominal surgery.

An abdominoplasty is an operation we do for people who have a particular concern for the appearance of their abdomen, in or out of clothing. Most people who decide to do it are pleased that they did it.

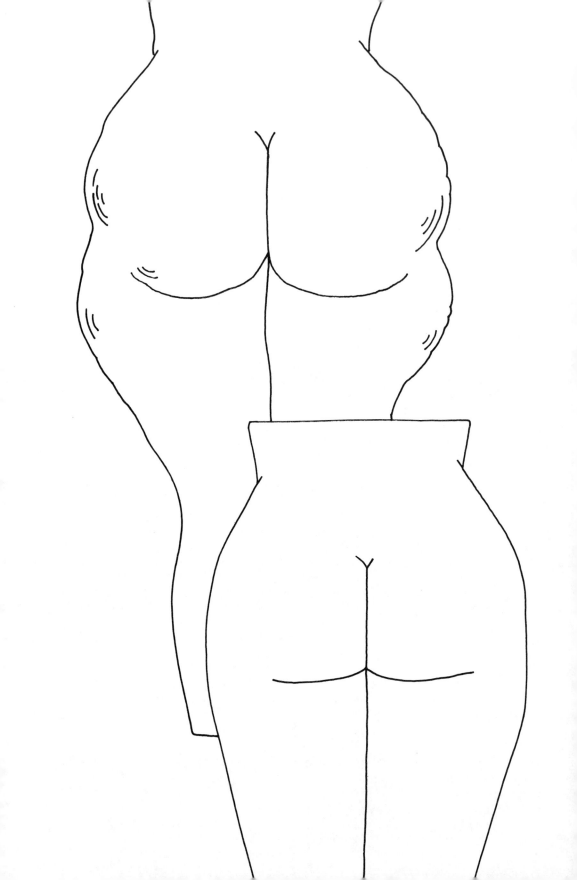

16

Liposuction, Lipoplasty, Lipolysis

In the early 1980's, plastic surgeons in France developed a technique to remove fat from beneath the skin through tiny incisions. This procedure involved using a powerful suction device with a long thin blunt tube that could pass in the areas of excess fat.

There followed an exodus of American plastic surgeons to Europe to learn how to use this new procedure. A number of separate societies of liposuction evolved in the U.S. Each society designed a certificate for the wall of the doctor's office, but the sophisticated shopper must look beyond these to determine the surgeon's qualifications. Liposuction is not difficult surgery to perform. As a result, many doctors who are not in surgical specialties have lurched into the field for purposes of profit. Liposuction requires judgment and experience to get quality results.

Liposuction does, as in all surgery, have complications, some even fatal--so it is important to find a surgeon who is qualified, and who also has access to facilities to deal with those complications. As patients rarely discuss their plan to have body sculpturing procedures with their family doctor, they are even more likely to find their sculptor through advertising for liposuction than they would for other aesthetic procedures.

Liposuction, lipolysis, fat suctioning, or lipoplasty, whatever it is called, is a favorite playground for fringe physicians who have more concern for their own financial gain than for the welfare of the unsophisticated patient. So, again, be a cautious buyer. Ask the receptionist about the doctor's credentials and experience. Find out if he has full surgical privileges in an approved hospital. How many liposuctions does he do each month? Is he one of the doctors that younger doctors come to to learn and to gain experience? Again, the question of advertising. If I look in the yellow pages of communities where the recognized sources of knowledge in liposuction practice, I'll generally find their names listed without any advertising at all.

The patient presents a problem to the surgeon which may or may not be best treated by liposuction alone.

If the liposucker has no surgical background, he is likely to recommend liposuction alone, where the best result would be obtained by a combination of liposuction and surgical sculpture, or by surgical sculpture alone--yet, another reason to select a plastic surgeon as your liposucker.

The use of liposuction has become a tool in surgery. It is used to remove fatty tumors, to reduce the size of arms swollen with lymphedema after radiation for breast cancer. It is used, in my practice, to remove the fat under the chin in face-lifting. It also has a place in making breasts the proper shape in breast reduction. Plastic surgeons have been doing procedures for many years to surgically contour body parts, removing both skin and fat. The abdomen, breasts, and less frequently the hips, thighs, and upper arms are principal subjects. The development of liposuction has had an effect on many of these. Often, the surgery is no longer appropriate and can be replaced by liposuction. More frequently, liposuction can improve the result of the the surgical procedure, and with this technique it need not be as extensive.

About Liposuction Surgery
Liposuction is, ideally, a method of removing excess deposits of fat from an individual who has unsightly fat deposits and who is at or near normal weight. Liposuction is ideal in the removal of the Jodhpur deformity some people have in the upper lateral thighs. It is also useful to reduce fat deposits in the sides of the abdomen, on the flanks, in fatty knees, and in the lower abdomen, where muscle tone is good and intra-abdominal fat isn't excessive. It can also reduce some modestly enlarged buttocks. It is not a proper substitute for weight reduction and should be considered a reward for successful weight reduction to top off the reduction with an improved contour.

Fat cells are thought to increase in size, rather than number when one gains weight. We believe that liposuction removes the fat cells, and, as a result, the local disproportion can be removed permanently if the offending fat cells are removed. This has not been proven, but it has not yet been questioned seriously.

The Procedure
Small amounts of liposuction can be done on an outpatient basis under local anesthesia. I prefer to limit this technique to a pound (500cc) or less of fat sucked. Larger amounts require a general anesthetic and careful fluid replacement during and after surgery. Liposuction makes a large wound in the space under the skin which can be compared to a burn in its biological needs. A significant amount of fluid is lost from the blood stream into the wound under the skin, so it is necessary to replace this fluid and its accompanying salts to keep a healthy blood volume. In extensive liposuction, autotransfusions are appropriate to replace the accompanying blood loss. (Autotransfusions are those where a patient gives blood for his own future use. It is rare, these days, to use another's blood for optional surgery in healthy patients.)

Many surgeons limit their liposuction to 2000 cc (2+ quarts) at a session, but this is not absolute and many patients have had considerably more removed in special situations. The more fat removed, the more complex the management of the patient. Obviously, if it is necessary to remove a large amount of fat, it is reasonable to suspect that the patient has refused to lose weight conventionally, or the surgeon is a little impatient to operate upon the patient rather than to serve the patient's needs.

Liposuction is done by passing a blunt steel tube with holes near its end, back and forth through an incision into the channel of fat under the skin. A very strong suction machine is attached to the tube through which the fat is sucked out and deposited in a bottle. The movement of the surgeon is much like a violinist using a bow. The incisions are small and usually heal quite inconspicuously. There are commonly two small incisions for each area of work. It is quite appropriate and customary to work on several sites--hips, abdomen, knees, etc., at a single procedure.

110

The result of the surgery is quite evident immediately after it is done, but often the patient doesn't see this early result because of the prompt onset of swelling. This swelling is greatest in the first few days and gradually diminishes. It is not completely gone until three or four months after surgery. Fortunately, the swelling rarely is larger than the preoperative condition after the first few days. Most patients are put in elastic garments over the liposuction areas for about 10 days after surgery.

After surgery, there is considerable bruising which may take several weeks to clear completely. The pain is annoying, but not usually severe, and it can be controlled by the usual oral postoperative medication. It is worse immediately after the operation and then gradually subsides. After a couple of days, it doesn't make much difference whether one is up and about, or in bed. Activity often makes the discomfort easier to tolerate, as boredom always makes it worse.

Complications
The serious complications of liposuction are rare, but they are complications of surgery which require surgical judgment, surgical skill, and occasionally surgery itself, to keep them under control. The sophisticated shopper wants to find a liposucker who is a qualified surgeon in addition to his experience and expertise in lipoplasty. This should not be difficult as there are many plastic surgeons who are fully trained and fully qualified.

Expectations
Liposuction does nothing significant for cellulite, and the removal of fat from under wrinkled skin often makes it look worse. Nonetheless, we do liposuction in the presence of cellulite or wrinkled skin with the understanding that the patient wants to look better in clothes, and can accept the fact that the result won't look great in the nude.

Cellulite, by the way, is the condition (seen typically in obese or oversized legs and buttocks) where there are numerous dents in the surface of the skin. These are the result of fibrous bands between the skin and the deeper structures which do not stretch enough with increasing fat, causing dimples in the fat-expanded skin. For reasons that are not clearly understood, reduction of fat by suction technique does not take them away. Some early attempts to cut these bands loose resulted in skin which would sag down like bloomers as a result of the lack of attachment to the underlying muscles.

The results of liposuction procedures are rarely perfect. Symmetry is impossible to achieve in the human body as no one is symmetrical. Surgeons try to avoid dents, ridges, and other irregularities, but they are impossible to completely avoid. Recently, it has become customary to use smaller liposuction instruments which can reduce the likelihood of dents and grooves. These make the procedure take a little longer, but the result is well worth it. Like all aesthetic procedures, occasionally the surgeon and patient will want to improve a result with a secondary touch-up procedure. Sometimes, liposuction procedures are planned in stages at different times.

The quality of the final product is dependent upon the skill of the surgeon and the material the patient provides for the surgeon's work. The happy patient is one who has an adequate result and has understood what to expect. Be sure your surgeon explains in detail what he intends to achieve, and what you are going to have to go through to get there. If he can't, or won't, you may want to find another surgeon. Aesthetic procedures are purely voluntary and the volunteer should be well informed of the costs, inconveniences, risks, pains, and expected benefits before he signs on.

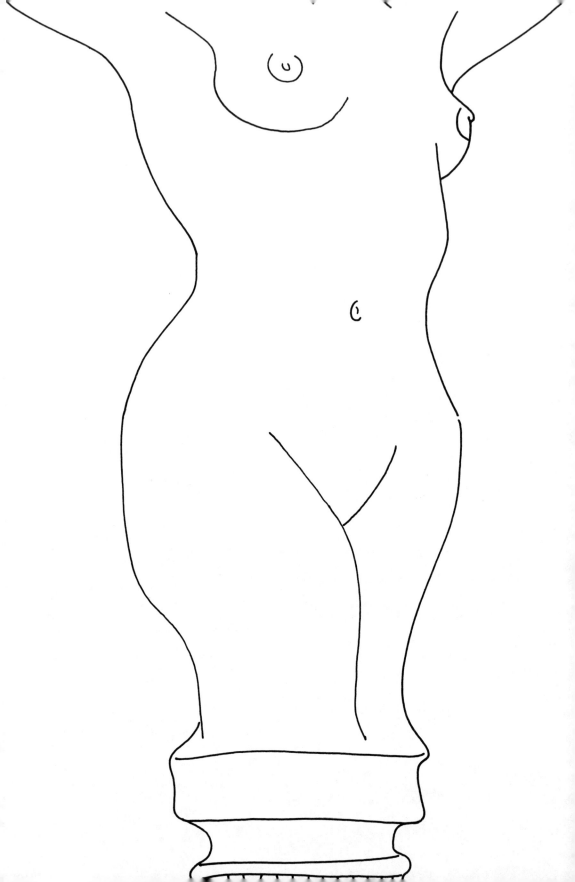

17

Other Body Sculpture Surgery

We have talked of reshaping breasts, noses, ears, chins, and tummies, but we haven't discussed all of the areas of the body that are reshaped, surgically, for aesthetic reasons.

The largest problems are found with the patients who get over great obesity, and have folds of excess skin to be removed. The inner thighs, the upper arms, and the buttock are frequently trimmed of skin and fat to improve the contour. These operations vary as the problems offered by patients are all different.

These surgeries commonly involve long incisions which do not scar very well. Customarily, large amounts of tissue is removed, and the scars are a welcome trade. Because of the amount of tissue removed, these operations are usually done under general anesthesia and both sides are usually done at once. Hospital stays are not long, as deeper structures are rarely involved; but, hospital stays are common.

Before liposuction was available, these operations were more common and more extensive. Now, many of the smaller body sculpture procedures are done with liposuction, particularly in younger women.

When body sculpture surgery is done, it is frequently accompanied by liposuction, either at the same time or during a separate procedure. With liposuction the size of the body sculpture operation is usually greatly reduced. Patients are grateful for this, as those who want their shape modified are understandably unenthusiastic about scars.

For cultural reasons that are little understood, body sculpture procedures to get rid of prominent hips, buttocks, and thighs occupy much more of the time and operative lists of our colleagues in Latin America. There women and men seem to be more concerned about the shapes of their torsos than the average citizens in the United States. Although recent enthusiasm for liposuction in the U.S. which has clearly resulted from lots of publicity, suggests that gringos may share this "cultural" propensity. The differences may be merely differences in marketing surgical services.

Patients who clearly understand the extent of possible scarring and who are willing to accommodate them in trade for a reduction in awkward prominences are almost always pleased with the result.

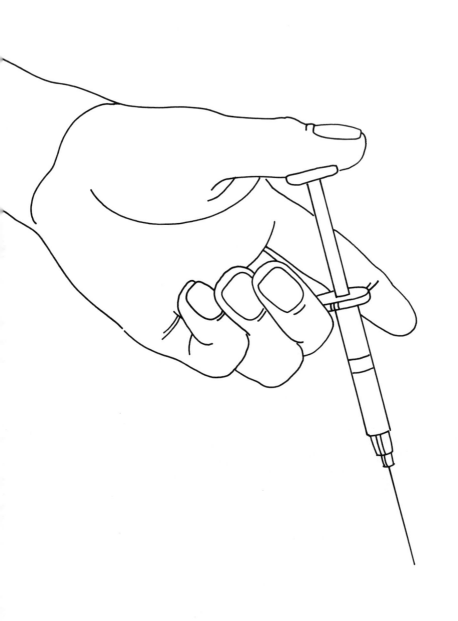

18

Collagen
And Other
Injectables

When silicone was first discovered to be an acceptable implant into mammalian tissues, it was tried in many forms. The injection of a fluid form of silicone was an obvious answer to many of the problems in reconstructive and aesthetic plastic surgery where fat in particular, had been lost from under the skin. As a result, silicone liquid was used in many situations as a new miraculous drug. It was injected into depressed scars, wrinkles, breasts, and into the peculiar anomalies of the human called hemifacial atrophy because it was an easy, inexpensive way to provide fill where it was needed.

Time demonstrated that injected silicone was not stable enough to provide an adequate substitute for what it was used to replace. It had a tendency to spread beyond the bounds of the defect into which it had been injected. It created tissue and foreign body reactions, which were lumpy and, in the breast, could not be easily distinguished from tumors. It infiltrated the skin and weakened it , causing ulcers. It even came out the ducts in the nipples.

As a result, the F.D.A. limited its use to a few selected plastic surgeons for special applications which do not include the breasts. Few of these surgeons use the material now.

The experience with silicone, the beautiful early results, and the ease with which it could be accomplished, has caused a continued search for something that is similar, but without adverse reactions.

The best alternatives are products of the Collagen Corporation in California which manufactures for injection, Zyderm and Zyplast, both composed of mammalian collagen. (Collagen is the name of the principal fibrous structure in mammals which makes up the strong fibers in the skin, the tendons, the fascia, the valves of the heart, the strength of vessel walls, the joints and hundreds of other definable things in the mammalian body.)

Injectable collagen is made from the skin of calves from which everything except the structural fiber has been removed along with the ends of the long polymer molecules which identify the species of the mammal and the individual from which it came. The resulting protein is the raw material of mammalian fibrous tissue without the markers that identify it immunologically in 99 percent of people. It can, therefore, be injected into depressions and wrinkles of patients who do not fail a skin test that must be done 30 days in advance of the injection.

Injectable collagen is useful for wrinkles and depressions that stand alone or are the early signs of aging, and for touch-up in the parts of the face that were not optimally handled in surgery for aging. In my practice, I use it mostly for these two categories of patients:1) the young beginning to have an occasional wrinkle, and 2) patients who have had a face- or brow-lift and who have a few lines that were outside of the area of benefit from the surgery.

Collagen is by no means the ideal product, but it is an excellent step in the right direction. It is so like natural scar tissue that it is absorbed and used by the body as excess scar is in the normal healing process. It is also effective for a long enough period of time that the patient will come back willingly for a reinjection when the original material has begun to fade away.

I find collagen, usually Zyplast (the more concentrated, cross-linked variety) particularly useful in the deep lines between the brows, the furrows in the lips, and in lessening the depth of the nasolabial creases that frame the mouth.

Plastic surgeons are grateful to the Collagen Corporation for bringing this product out and advertising it so well to the public, because patients come into their offices who are not candidates for collagen injections, but need aesthetic surgery to solve the problem they thought collagen might help. It is unfortunate that collagen injections are available to doctors who don't understand the proper management of the problems of aging, and are unfamiliar with other, more appropriate forms of treatment.

It is generally known to more experienced plastic

surgeons that collagen is frequently injected into patients who would be better served by proper aesthetic surgical procedures. Usually, such patients are not offered the alternative, either because the injector doesn't know about the proper treatment, or does not wish to lose the patient.

Fat Injections

The ability to suck fat from one part of the body (liposuction) and inject it into another needy area of the body has been met with much enthusiasm in the plastic surgical field. To the best of my knowledge, there has been no evidence that this fat grafting can be depended upon to last. Much has been said about it as a technique, but little evidence has been presented that such fat will stay put. It appears to liquify and be absorbed by the normal biochemical processes of healing.

It is unwise to have such fat injections placed into the breast as it results in lumps that can not be easily distinguished from tumors. These fatty lumps also present problems in diagnosis on mammograms, as such injected fat promotes calcification, similar to that of breast tumors.

Periodically, someone comes up with yet another substance to be injected. For now, I can only suggest caution to the sophisticated shopper unless the shopper wishes to join the ranks of experimental animals.

19

How To Find Your Plastic Surgeon

The outcome of your plastic surgery adventure depends on your selection of the surgeon who does the work. He must be qualified, experienced and compatible if you're to get a good result and look back favorably on the experience.

In this book, we have dwelt heavily on the problems arising from doctors who do plastic surgery, but are not plastic surgeons. We must now help you to find a surgeon who is likely to serve you well.

A real plastic surgeon has had training exclusively directed toward a full time plastic surgical career. He is able to discuss all aspects of your plastic surgical needs. His training in plastic surgery has been his primary focus and not a small part of the training in another field such as ear, nose and throat, dermatology, or ophthalmology.

The molding of tissues to fit a problem or a desire which is the essence of all plastic surgery, and the derivation of the word "plastic," is not unique to one part of the body. Experience all over the body lends a basis for proper decisions for any particular problem. A plastic surgeon must be able to choose from many alternatives to arrive at the best approach to your problem. We don't want a surgeon who uses a particular method for all of his patients, as the method will fit only some of them best.

Most of the plastic surgeons in our country have certain credentials which the sophisticated shopper should look for. If you are checking the credentials of, or looking for, a plastic surgeon, there are several ways to go about it. Some of these are discussed in the chapter called "Clubs."

Directories

Board Certification in plastic surgery can be investigated in several ways. Many public libraries have a Directory of Medical Specialists put out by Marquis Who's Who Inc., or the Compendium of Certified Medical Specialists kept up-to-date by the American Board of Medical Specialists, the mother organization of American Medical Specialty Boards. These Boards are the established, accepted Specialty Boards which respect the existence of each other and measure each other's criteria. There are other self-proclaimed boards which will not, or have not subjected themselves to this scrutiny. Some, with very classy names, are for the sole purpose of documenting less well-trained individuals as plastic surgeons. These large directories have geographical listings, so you can look up your town or city and see who is listed there. The biographical listings will also tell you which clubs the surgeon belongs to which is a further guide.

Ask The Doctor
The receptionist in any plastic surgeon's office will tell you which board he is certified by. Beware, though, "Board Certified Plastic Surgeon" usually means that the surgeon wishes to be regarded as a plastic surgeon when he has been trained in another field. Ask which board certified the doctor.

Ask about society (club) membership. Many sound alike so listen carefully. The ones you want to hear about are: The American Society of Plastic and Reconstructive Surgeons, The American Society of Aesthetic Plastic Surgeons, The American Association of Plastic Surgeons, The Lipoplasty Society, and some regional societies of plastic surgeons like, the California Society of Plastic Surgeons. There are many others that sound right, but they don't have the stringent membership requirements. If it sounds like the person answering the phone is hedging, you would be wise to call someone else.

Hospital/County Medical Society
Hospital staff offices and county medical societies know the qualifications of all members and can be expected to answer questions about qualifications, or give recommended lists of real plastic surgeons. Again, you must be specific and ask for full-time plastic surgeons, or for those who are certified by the American Board of Plastic Surgeons.

The American Society of Plastic And Reconstructive Surgeons

One may contact the American Society of Plastic and Reconstructive Surgeons at 1-800/635-0635, or the California Society of Plastic Surgeons at 1-800/722-2777. If you tell the operator what you want done, he or she will send you a list of professionals in your community who are qualified and have an interest in your type of case.

Ask Your Doctor?

Remember that your doctor may know less about the training and qualifications of a real plastic surgeon than you do.

Ask The Plastic Surgeon Himself?

I feel it a sign of sophistication and intelligence when a patient asks me about my experience or my training. If this question creates a defensive response in your prospective plastic surgeon, it is time to look further.

Don't expect a plastic surgeon to show you his own results. Many plastic surgeons won't show you examples of their own work for two reasons. First, there is a concern that you might know the patient, and the surgeon will have invaded a patient's privacy. Second, we are human and are likely to be reluctant to show anything except our very best results, when we have no assurance that you will be a best result. Even those of us who feel this way will show pictures of breast reconstructions and other problems when the patient identity is not a problem and the potential patient needs to know the limitations of our work. Be a little wary of the surgeon who only shows his best results.

Fees

You should be able to get some approximation of a surgeon's fees in discussion with the office staff, but the final determination will depend on what the surgeon feels you need done, and what you agree to have done. For aesthetic/cosmetic surgery, fees are customarily paid in advance.

Fees for aesthetic surgery vary widely, depending upon the region and what the traffic will bear. There is little relationship between the fee and the quality of the result. This goes both ways. Surgeons, essentially without training or experience, will charge the same prices as the more experienced surgeons in the community, and surgeons who charge very high fees don't generally out-perform their peers.

Insurance

Reconstructive plastic surgery is usually covered by insurance, though there is often a fight to get coverage. Aesthetic operations are generally not covered. Insurance companies have extensive experience with all the games that have been tried to get coverage for cosmetic surgery, so it is futile to attempt to get them to bend the rules. A WARNING: Some insurance companies exclude coverage of the complications of aesthetic surgery. So, if you are one of the rare people who have a severe complication, it can become quite expensive.

Your Contact With The Plastic Surgeon -
The Consultation

Your final decision will occur after you have seen the surgeon. At the consultation you will learn what the surgeon will do for you, whether he listens carefully, whether he shows interest in your problem, and whether you want to begin a relationship with this person and his staff.

The time in the consultation will be better spent if you have an idea what it is you expect to achieve. It will be helpful if you have read a bit about what you have in mind. Your questions will be better organized.

Your surgeon should have an interest in your reasons for your concern about your problem as well as the problem itself. He should be willing to discuss fees and the details of the surgical plan with you. He should not pressure you for a decision. He should welcome questions about his experience and qualifications. He should answer your questions openly, and volunteer information about the complications and hazards of the treatment contemplated. If there are alternate methods of treatment, he should explain his reasons for choosing what he recommends. He should not promise you anything.

If your consultation doesn't feel right, you should consider seeing someone else. It is better not to tell the second or third surgeon about the earlier ones, as the doctor will be more at ease if he doesn't think he is being compared.

In plastic surgery, we often use pamphlets or visual aids to assist in educating our patients. Sometimes even modifying the patient's profile, etc., on a video screen. Such information should be presented as a guide only. Even the video modifications cannot be an accurate portrayal of a final result.

It is unfortunate that all this is necessary preparation for your embarkation into the world of plastic surgery, but the decision is important and the sophisticated shopper should be well-informed.

INDEX

E
ears
>correction of, 68-69
>complications, 69
>postoperative pain, 69
>prominent, 68-69

Elephant Man Disease, 40
endocrinologist, 32
estrogen, 31, 32
expanders, 73, 81, 94, 96

F
face-lift, 30-40
>aging process, 30-32
>ambulatory surgery, 35
>anesthesia for, 34-35
>complications, 36
>disapointments, 35
>liposuction and, 40
>nerve injury, 36
>other complimenting procedures, 38
>repeated, 37-38
>SMAS, 33-34
>what is a, 32-33

facial plastic surgeon, 5
fat
>grafting, 122
>injections, 122

FDA, 78, 79
Federal Trade Commission, 15
fees, 126-127
fibrosarcoma, 79

G
gynecologist, 32
gynecology, 9

mucous membranes, 31

N
National Geographic, 86
navel, 102
neurofibromatosis, 40
nipple reconstruction, 97
nose job *(see rhinoplasty)*, 52

O
obstetrics, 9
oculoplastic surgeon, 5
ophthalmologist, 21
Orentreich, Norman, 73
orthodontist, 21, 22, 62, 64
otoplasty, 68
otorhinolaryngology, 9, 21, 52

P
Pegram, Max, 30
pituitary gland, 62
polyvinyl sponges, 78
PPOs, 17
professional behavior, 10, 15-17
Proplast, 39, 63
psychiatrist, 25
pulmonary emboli, 104

R
referrals, 9, 10, 83
rhinoplasty, 52-58
      bleeding, 56
      infection, 56
      operation, the, 54-56
      pain, 56
      secondary surgery, 57
      septum, 57
rhytidectomy, 32